WALKING YOUR TALK

WALKING YOUR TALK

ALSO BY LAVINIA PLONKA

What Are You Afraid Of?
A Body/Mind Guide to Courageous Living

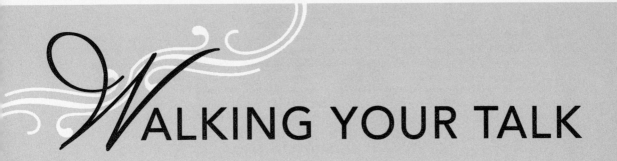

WALKING YOUR TALK

Changing Your Life Through the
Magic of Body Language

LAVINIA PLONKA

JEREMY P. TARCHER/PENGUIN

a member of Penguin Group (USA) Inc.

New York

JEREMY P. TARCHER/PENGUIN
Published by the Penguin Group
Penguin Group (USA) Inc., 375 Hudson Street, New York, New York 10014, USA • Penguin Group (Canada), 90 Eglinton
Avenue East, Suite 700, Toronto, Ontario M4P 2Y3, Canada (a division of Pearson Penguin Canada Inc.) • Penguin Books Ltd,
80 Strand, London WC2R 0RL, England • Penguin Ireland, 25 St Stephen's Green, Dublin 2, Ireland (a division of Penguin
Books Ltd) • Penguin Group (Australia), 250 Camberwell Road, Camberwell, Victoria 3124, Australia (a division of Pearson
Australia Group Pty Ltd) • Penguin Books India Pvt Ltd, 11 Community Centre, Panchsheel Park, New Delhi–110 017,
India • Penguin Group (NZ), 67 Apollo Drive, Mairangi Bay, Auckland 1311, New Zealand (a division of Pearson
New Zealand Ltd) • Penguin Books (South Africa) (Pty) Ltd, 24 Sturdee Avenue, Rosebank, Johannesburg 2196, South Africa

Penguin Books Ltd, Registered Offices:
80 Strand, London WC2R 0RL, England

Most Tarcher/Penguin books are available at special quantity discounts for bulk purchase for sales promotions, premiums, fund-
raising, and educational needs. Special books or book excerpts also can be created to fit specific needs. For details, write Penguin
Group (USA) Inc. Special Markets, 375 Hudson Street, New York, NY 10014.

Library of Congress Cataloging-in-Publication Data

Plonka, Lavinia.
Walking your talk: changing your life through the magic of body language / Lavinia Plonka.
p.   cm.
Includes bibliographical references and index.
ISBN 978-1-58542-542-6
1. Body language.   I. Title.
BF637.N66P55   2007   2006037108
153.6'9—dc22

Printed in the United States of America
1   3   5   7   9   10   8   6   4   2

Book design by Meighan Cavanaugh

ACKNOWLEDGMENTS

This book would not be possible without the hundreds of students who have shared their stories, taken risks, and participated in countless movement experiments. I am also indebted to all my teachers—the list would take pages, and each one has shone another light on my path. I would like to personally thank Laura Facciponti for her help in researching the Alba Emoting Method. Alan Questel, one of Feldenkrais's original U.S. students and a Feldenkrais trainer, mentored me throughout the project. Richard Lipton pressed the crumbling copy of *Delsartes System of Expression* into my hands one day, saying simply, "I think you might get some use out of this." Mitch Horowitz, my editor at Tarcher/Penguin, has a keen eye and an elegant approach to writing that clarified my prose immeasurably. And to all of the workshop sponsors and organizers around the country who have dedicated time and energy to bringing this work to their communities—I thank you.

CONTENTS

Part Two

Experience

Part Three
Synthesis

Ten
PRACTICAL SHAPE-SHIFTING

Eleven
EMBODYING COMPASSION

WALKING YOUR TALK

WALKING YOUR TALK

INTRODUCTION

ARE YOU WHO YOU SAY YOU ARE?

You go for a job interview and you think it went well, only to find that you didn't get the job. You envy someone surrounded by a group of enthralled admirers at a party where you can't seem to get a conversation started. While walking down a street, you pass a couple of men. Hearing a scream, you turn and see them grab a woman's purse and run off. Why her and why not you? Is there something in the way you walk, stand, and act that affects others?

Often people say one thing and do another. They desire something, then unconsciously sabotage it. They begin with an intention and then find themselves at cross purposes. Dreams and wishes seem to get waylaid by life's circumstances so that existence becomes "a life of quiet desperation." Is it possible that even your successes and failures in life have something to do with your carriage, your walk, your gestures—and not just the words you say? Body language affects everything—your relationships, your potency, your self image. These in turn affect your happiness, personal power, and, ultimately, your health.

Back pain, sexual impotence, immune and anxiety disorders, headaches, and much more can often be traced back to how you use your body every moment of your life. You are not just communicating with others; you are constantly communicating with your entire organism. Your clenched jaw, gripped buttocks, jutting chin affect other people even as they are affecting your nervous system, skeletal organization, and the circulation of your blood.

Many body language books focus on reading others: how to know when someone's lying, who is the right woman for you, and so on. Others offer body language tips for business success: how to close a sale or land the right job. I propose a deeper study—your own body language, wherein you will discover the possibility of how to literally change your life.

ANY-BODY HOME?

Ask the average person if he is aware of himself and chances are he'll scoff (slightly dilated nostrils, pulling nose upward in a signal of dismissal, head moving back slightly in a gesture of rejection as eyebrows come up and toward center in disbelief) and say, "Of course I am!" But if you ask him to tell you what his body just did in reaction to your question, he'll be unable to answer.

We all have an invisible sixth sense—the kinesthetic sense. Our kinesthetic sense is what teaches us how to ride a bike, gives us our spatial orientation and our ability to recognize a friend or foe. Yet we are as unaware of this process as a fish is of water. Most of our lives are spent oblivious to kinesthetic habits and reactions that are constantly affecting our attitudes, perceptions, and behavior. Many are essential. You don't want to have to think when avoiding an oncoming car or about how to chop an onion. Yet even in these moments a whole world of emotional expression exists. Most of the time we are driven by unconscious triggers, yet are unaware of much of what is taking place. The thoughts run on, emotions churn, the body tenses and relaxes, movement is sometimes elegant, sometimes awkward.

Awareness of this kinesthetic sense could be called embodiment, literally living in the body. By experiencing fully what takes place in standing, walking, talking, making love, or fighting, it's possible not only to attain what you want in the world—financial success, creative fulfillment, or healthy relationships—but you can also become a different person by understanding and transforming the tool with which you chiefly, and unknowingly, engage the world.

MOVEMENT IS MY LIFE

This book is the result of a thirty-year journey, beginning with a career in theater. As a movement specialist and choreographer, I was trained in the classical arts of mime, commedia dell'arte, and many forms of dance, from ballet to Kathakali. I studied physical acting techniques from all over the world—rigorous training programs designed to make an actor's body a finely tuned instrument. Many years teaching both theater and yoga to diverse populations, from professional actors to at-risk children in the inner city, afforded me a magnificent laboratory for the study of human expression.

Yet there were so many mysteries that begged further investigation. For example, as you're standing on a corner your eye catches someone walking a couple of blocks away. It's a friend you haven't seen in five years. Even at that distance you recognize him from his walk, his carriage. How? Why? What is the relationship between the way we organize our posture, our physical bearing, and the way we organize our lives? Why do some people seem trustworthy, confident, and others give us the creeps? What does it have to do with the habitual postural choices we make every second? I wondered how my own choices interfered with what I wanted to accomplish in life. I began to question how much of what I call "me" was just a collection of habits learned from my parents, education, and society.

At that point I discovered a field called somatic education: literally learning through movement. After exploring several different approaches, I enrolled in a Feldenkrais Professional Training Program in 1990. Much of the information in this book is indebted to this elegant method of learning, which was developed by Dr. Moshe Feldenkrais, which I will explain in depth as the book unfolds. The training provided me the opportunity to study on a microcosmic level the relationship between each movement and my experience of myself.

When I opened my practice, generally people would come to see me as a last resort. Feldenkrais is not a household word; for many it's hard even to pronounce. It's not covered by most health insurance. So I received the desperate, the cynical, the hopeless. Almost everyone who came had physical pain—due to injury, illness, or just some undiagnosable discomfort that defied medicine. My students and I discovered the deep relationships between their pain and the movement habits they'd developed over the course of their lives. Even people with permanent physical damage due to accidents, birth defects, or stroke learned that their particular approach to their physical challenges affected their development.

When people come into my office I don't see a collection of symptoms to be dissected and repaired. Instead, I see a story about to unfold. The defiant little boy who at age fifty-nine is still daring his parents to say no. The successful executive who still shields her face from the blows she received from her alcoholic father twenty years ago. The twelve-year-old girl with scoliosis who has no idea what it's like to stand up for herself. We don't work psychologically; we work directly with the physical habits. Slowly the story emerges, sometimes in words, sometimes in an elegant reorganization of the posture that makes words extraneous. Suddenly a young man who always walks on his toes has his heels on the ground. He is more confident, more balanced. Another man's chest has become softer, it is not jutting out and frozen, forcing his arms to move separately from the skeleton and creating shoulder injuries. He realizes he no longer has to protect himself from jeering high school peers.

Throughout this book we will study the stories that have emerged from this work. While the stories in this book are all based on work with my students, I have made every effort to protect their confidentiality. I have retained the relevant material, while changing all personal details. It is my hope that through these examples, you will recognize your own story. Many times I will focus on one aspect of an individual's body language in order to illustrate a concept, but understand that each person is infinitely more complex than the few characteristics I examine in a particular chapter. The truth is that each person I work with contains a story so rich in his walk, her posture, his gesture, her face, that to truly do them justice, they'd each merit a book of their own.

Feldenkrais himself often said that pure physical rehabilitation was not his aim. Instead, it was to help others "realize their avowed and unavowed dreams." He defined unavowed dreams as the waylaid intentions and ambitions of our childhood. We give up these dreams, blaming circumstance, fear, society, or injury. They get buried under myths of security and responsibility and our posture then reflects this. Compulsions arise that forbid spontaneity, risk taking, and freedom of choice. Eventually walking your talk is no longer an issue, because you've long ago forgotten about that screenplay you were going to write, the trip to India you had planned, or the pilot's license you had dreamed of. My hope here is to reawaken for you the possibility of reconnecting with that sense of joyful possibility. By understanding your physical "instant messages" you can begin to uncover the potency and vitality within yourself and be the person you say you are.

HOW TO USE THIS BOOK

This is a workbook. Every chapter contains both information and exercises and explorations that can begin to awaken your innate kinesthetic abilities. I have found it extremely useful to have a journal or notebook in which to collect the information and impressions that the exercises offer, although there are as many ways to record information as there are styles of learning. I've had students record their input on their MP3s, use their insights to create colorful drawings, make flow charts complete with arrows and circles, and write on loose-leaf paper and add it to a binder along with materials from other sources. How or whether you choose to record your insights is up to you.

The book is designed to guide you through the territory known as yourself; to be absorbed not just with the mind, the way we normally read, but to include an inner, kinesthetic experience that allows for physiological and psychological change. Some exercises can be done alone; others need other people. After all, the study of body language requires that we look beyond the pages of a book.

While it is tempting to just read the book through, I invite you to use the format of this book as an opportunity to break out of your habitual approach to learning. Take some time each day, each week, to explore the physical exercises offered. While some are easily folded into the course of the day, some will require that you find a quiet space, to lie down, to take up to a half hour to explore a movement pattern or habit. If you need to skip over a section because you are reading the book on the subway or in the employee cafeteria, take the time when you get home to go back and try the sequence. Many of these exercises are done in a space on the floor. Perhaps your living situation or a physical disability does not allow complete freedom of movement—you can still do variations of the exercises by keeping them small or by imagining the sequences that are not possible to execute. If space is the limitation, however, I highly recommend you explore the possibility of creating a "movement exploration" space in your home.

We have become so divorced from a true relationship with this two-legged creature that carries our thoughts and feelings around that we actually think we know how it works, what it does. This couldn't be further from the truth. Only by intently listening to yourself *while* engaged in movement will be you begin to understand your personal incongruities and learn to truly walk your talk.

While working through this book might seem like an investment, I guarantee that if you dedicate yourself to the process, you will never look at anyone, including yourself, in the same way again.

Part One

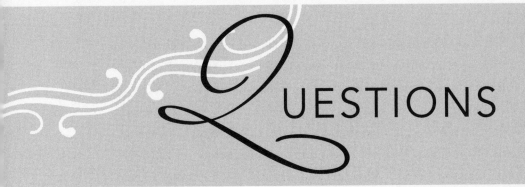

QUESTIONS

*A*ll investigation begins with a question—something you wish to know. For myself, it is a continuous quest for a deeper understanding of who I am. But the nature of the question changes. Sometimes it's big—"Why am I here?" Sometimes it seems petty—"Why doesn't he like me?" Sometimes there is a recurrence, a question that returns in a different form or strength at points of my life—"Why do I abandon a project before it's finished?" "Why do I hate parties?" " Why can't I make money at the things I love?" Before you go further, I invite you to record some of your questions at this moment. They may change while you're working through this book. They may seem to have nothing to do with body language right now. They may seem dumb. But it's the beginning of our investigation.

This first section introduces you to some of the ideas and theories behind the work you will be undertaking, preparing you for the questioning process that you will practice throughout the book.

One

AM I WALKING MY TALK?

Fie, fie upon her!
There's language in her eye, her cheek, her lip,
Nay, her foot speaks;
her wanton spirits look out
At every joint and motive of her body.

William Shakespeare, *Troilus and Cressida*

Your body is talking all the time—whether you want it to or not. Even if you choose to sit absolutely still, you still are communicating. The way you choose to sit still, your alignment, various tensions, your facial expression, are all part of the story. Every activity is filled with information: how you hold the knife as you slice an onion, for example. It tells someone whether you love cooking, hate onions, or are afraid of knives. You'll slice differently after making love, after having a fight with a parent, or while anxiously waiting for a phone call about your tardy child. The way you bend over the chopping board may be the way your mother bent over the board as she chopped. Your stance may be the result, or the cause, of back pain, which is also visible to an attentive observer. While it's important to learn how your body communicates to others, what is more useful is the information you can gather for your own development. Your every move can serve as a feedback device that informs you of your emotional state, your intentions, your health, and your attention. Over the course of your day—with the people you encounter or in your moments alone—there is a universe of information at your fingertips, with every breath, each turn of the head that is waiting for you.

When I begin teaching people, sometimes they'll just sigh in exasperation. "Oh my gosh, there is so much to observe! I'm exhausted." The feeling of being overwhelmed at the sheer complexity and subtlety of the levels with which the body speaks can seem truly astronomical. After all, we have spent our lives ignoring our bodies' signals—to our detriment. It almost feels as if there's been an insidious conspiracy to convince us that there is nothing to listen to. From abhorrence of the body's functions and desires, by certain religions, to the endless distractions provided by entertainment media and drugs, to the mechanistic theories that prevailed in science and medicine since Descartes, we have treated the body like a stupid apparatus that is either ruled by our mental will or absolutely out of control. An example of this disassociation is the practice of working out at a gym while watching TV or reading—as if the physical body and mind have nothing to do with each other.

Baron von Münchhausen was a German nobleman known for his tall tales. In one of his adventures he travels to the moon, where the king and queen of the moon have the ability to separate their heads from their body—so that the bodies can be engaged in one activity while the head is doing something else. The poor king is so ashamed of his body's appetites, and of how his body controls him when it is attached to his head, that he tries to remove himself permanently from his body, even trying to destroy it in order to free himself. But it is only when he is united with his body that he can truly feel emotion.

Imagine living your life never having used your eyes, so in effect you are blind but don't know it. One day someone points out to you that what you call seeing has nothing to do with seeing by using your eyes. For a brief moment your eyes clear and you are able to see a fragment of a tree. But then it's immediately gone and within minutes you forget what it was like. Eventually you convince yourself that it was just a dream. That of course you know how to "see." But evidence mounts up that you are missing something. You can't forget what you have "seen." You realize you must stop lying to yourself about what you see. And it becomes clear that in order to be able to see consistently, you have to practice. You have to pay attention. And then, one day, you are really seeing. You have developed your sense of sight. And what a payoff!

Our kinesthetic sense is the same. We think we know what we are doing, but it's really just our habits. In order to be able to "see" how we are, we have to develop a new way of looking or, rather, sensing. This process can be invigorating and empowering rather than frustrating. A musician is passionate about developing his sense of hearing. An artist sees color and nuance that most of us miss. Developing the kinesthetic sense enhances everything—from touching a doorknob to knowing when someone is lying, from improved reaction time to personal attractiveness.

GETTING TO KNOW ME

Christine was a perky, fit step aerobics instructor. When I asked her why she wanted a lesson, she said, "Well, my friends say I limp."

"Do you limp?"

"I don't know. It doesn't feel like I limp. Sometimes when I'm walking down the street I try to look in the shop windows to see if I limp, but it's hard to look and walk at the same time."

"Do you have any pain?"

"I don't think so."

An interesting answer—her disconnect was so complete she didn't "think" she could "feel" pain. When I asked Christine to walk, I saw she had a pronounced limp. She was hiking the right side of her pelvis up, shortening her ribs, and in effect shortening the right leg. This created a kind of clunk with each step. There was no point in pointing out the limp, since her friends had already failed at that. So we began to work together to explore the movement of her pelvis and ribs on each side. Slowly, by drawing her attention to how she used parts of herself, her story began to unfold—one of a determined woman who considered herself unattractive. She once had been extremely overweight and had gotten into aerobics in order to reclaim her life. Christine burned off her calories and burned her way into a fitness career. Still terrified of relationships, she spent all her time either working out or teaching classes, perfecting her body in order to compensate for her perceived ugliness.

Slowly her torso lengthened as she loosened her grip on her right side. Her face began to soften, and then one day she confessed that teaching aerobics was really painful, but she was afraid to give it up. She would have no job, she would get fat again, and lose all her friends. All of these fears had exacerbated the stress she was putting on her body with the pounding workouts.

Why she chose to grip on the right is not important—in fact, there were many possible reasons. An old hip injury, being right-handed, her tendency to tilt her head to the right, her habit of always stepping on the stairs in class with the right leg first—the list goes on and on. As the possibility for real change appeared, Christine disappeared, calling to tell me that her work schedule had changed and she could no longer make the drive to lessons.

Each one of us has habits and attitudes that are hidden in plain sight. Fears, injuries, and patterns from childhood form our unique physical characteristics. Without awareness of how we are, it is impossible to truly "walk the talk," since the talk doesn't know what the walk is doing!

Christine was in essence lying to herself and to others; she also was accepting limitations out of fear. These are just two examples of how our walk and talk come into conflict. Incongruence between words and actions is written in both gesture and action. Body language communicates to both ourselves and others. What occurs in your body as you reach for the phone to make that call? What happens physiologically when you change your mind and postpone the call till tomorrow yet again? Why do you lose your voice every time you go to an audition? Does having your fists clenched while talking to your boss get you the raise? How does it affect him? How does it affect your behavior? What do you think your spouse feels when you say I love you but your eyes are looking at a notice posted on the refrigerator and your arms are hanging by your sides?

FINDING NEUTRAL

There is no such thing, really, as an absolutely neutral posture. We are constantly shifting and reacting to circumstances around ourselves. In our culture good posture seems to mean shoulders back, belly in, head high. However, that implies that posture is a static state. One could say that really good organization of the body allows movement in any direction in response to any stimulus. All parts are available: the head to turn freely, the legs to move under the trunk, the trunk able to bend and stretch, and so on. Most of us have postural habits that limit free range of movement. The bowed head, the rounded back, the frozen pelvis, all create limitations.

In an acting workshop I taught recently I stated that each one of us has a unique and recognizable walk. Sarah raised her hand. "I don't see how anybody can judge me from my walk. My walk is just neutral; I'm not doing anything special." The entire class burst into laughter. Sarah's walk was anything but neutral. She thrust out her ample chest, her arms swinging behind her like a Chinese emperor swaying his long sleeves. Her hips echoed the movement of her arms, and she periodically added in a toss of her tousled hair. She was the embodiment of a sassy, brassy babe. Several members of the class volunteered to do Sarah's walk, including a couple of men. The shock of recognition made her blush but acknowledge that indeed she was far from neutral.

Before you can begin to study what happens in life encounters, you have to have a sense of what your personal neutral is. Even if you feel you know yourself, take a moment to go stand in front of a full-length mirror. Take a mental snapshot of the whole of yourself. Don't judge ("I look like a dork." "Look at that double chin!" "My posture is terrible."). Instead, just take note—in fact you literally can take notes. How do you look at yourself? What do you see? How do you stand? What does it feel like to leave your arms at your sides? Where do your hands want to go? What parts of you are centered? Aligned? What are you doing with your face? Turn your body to see your profile. It's hard to look at yourself completely while in profile, but just try to check it out and note your impressions about how you stand.

Now step away from the mirror and stand comfortably with your eyes closed. If standing with your eyes closed makes you dizzy, leave your eyes open but unfocused. Imagine there's a plumb line going through from the top of your head to the floor. At the bottom of this line is a little weight to keep the line in place. Some people will locate this line going through the center of the head and straight down; others will send it down the center of the body. Either way is okay. Now notice where your head is in relation to your line. Don't try to correct anything during this exercise—just notice. Is it bisected by the line? Forward? Backward? Slightly right or left? Where are your shoulders? Are they symmetrical? How does the line go through your chest? Is your pelvis in front of the line or behind? Are both hips on the same level? As you follow the string to the floor, notice the relation of the string to your feet. Perhaps the string is a little closer to one foot or a little backward or forward. Just notice.

It's important not to change anything, for a number of reasons. First of all, as mentioned earlier, your perceptions are based on your habits. Until you truly know how and why you are feeling this, any attempt to change will just create more tension in the body. Just beginning to really *know* how you stand is a big exercise. And to do it without judgment is extremely challenging.

You may have noticed that things are not necessarily neatly lined up. Or that you get tense when trying to scan yourself in this way. Or you may have noticed absolutely nothing. All of these observations are valid and important, including noticing that you don't notice. The ability to distinguish differences in anything requires practice. An experienced chef can taste a dish and know exactly how much of a spice is missing in order to make the dish perfect. An artist senses the difference between carmine and scarlet in a way that the ordinary eye might miss. So it is with the art of noticing the self.

A POSTURAL AUTOBIOGRAPHY

If you have access to photos or videos of yourself throughout your life, take an evening to go through them. See if there is any information in them that can inform your current observations.

Lynette came to me with sore feet. Her gait was extremely stiff and tentative. Her knees were locked back and she had severe lower back pain. She wondered if some of the pain came from her years of being a marathon runner. She informed me that her coach in high school had taught her to run without moving her torso, pumping her legs while holding her pelvis and shoulders in place. Lynette felt that this habit had spilled into the rest of her life.

When we looked at photos of her as a child, it became clear that something had happened somewhere between the ages of three and four—long before she began her running career. At first there is a happy, relaxed little girl. Then suddenly she's standing at attention, knees locked back, a worried expression on her face. Lynette admitted that she was never good at any sports until she found running—it was clear why.

It was unimportant why Lynette developed these postures—the fact was that her rigidity was reflected in her career choices, her lack of relationships, her conservative attitudes. As she freed her pelvis, her back and knees relaxed. As her physical posture changed, so did her personality. She learned that she could move in many directions—both physically and emotionally.

Your personal neutral tells a story to everyone who sees you. You may not be able to see anything out of the ordinary as you study your photographs and videos. Like Sarah and her swinging walk, your posture and walking *are you.* This next exercise will help you begin to clarify your sense of proportion and your relationship to your plumb line.

The Cardinal Lines

Read through the instructions in this exercise before beginning. Lie down on your back, your legs stretched out, your arms horizontally out to the side. You may feel a bit like the famous Leonardo da Vinci illustration of the proportions of a man. And for good reason. Da Vinci's understanding of the symmetrical organization of the human body has proven to be true for most people. Da Vinci observed that the distance from fingertip to fingertip equals the distance of the head to toe.

Take a moment to picture the center of yourself. Where is center to you? In your abdomen? Solar plexus? From this center point, extend your attention down to the bottom of your pelvis, then up through the top of your head. Sense its direction—is it straight up and down, or does it angle to the right or left? Perhaps it changes directions a few times on its journey. Draw another line from right hip to your right foot. Sense the length of your leg. Imagine the direction of the line. Then do the same thing with your other leg. Above your torso, at the bottom of your neck, is a vertebra that may seem larger than the rest. For some people it is very prominent, for others not. But if your arms were extended horizontally and you drew a line from one arm to the other, this vertebra, known as your seventh cervical vertebra, would be in the middle of this line. Draw a line from your C7 down your right arm, and then your left. It's not important that all the lines are equal—some people have long legs and short arms, for example. What is more important is to note the relative distances between one arm and the other, the sense of how the line from your head to your center travels, and even the directions your lines point to. Many exercises in this book begin with a scan. Scanning while lying down informs you of certain habitual ways of holding or organizing yourself that may have something to do with how you are when you're standing and moving through life. People often don't notice differences in the beginning, or they have trouble imagining them in their mind's eye. If that's the case, let it go and return to the exercise at another time. It will get easier. As you continue working you will also notice shifts in the relationships along the cardinal lines.

Many times people tell me that when they first encounter these exercises they don't try them all in order, doing what attracts them and returning later on. For this reason at the end of each chapter I've included a checklist of the exercises covered. You can then quickly scan the exercises to see if there's one that attracts you today that you may have skipped, or one that you really valued and would like to repeat.

Exploration Checklist

- ☐ Check yourself out in the mirror.
- ☐ Study your postural relationship to the plumb line down the center of your body.
- ☐ Discover your postural history through pictures and videos.
- ☐ Explore the cardinal lines while lying down.

Two

NOT WALKING THE TALK

A man is never more truthful than when
he acknowledges himself as a liar.

MARK TWAIN

A menacing smile, crocodile tears, an air of bravado are some our descriptions of conflicting body signals. When someone is insincere, some part of you senses the tension behind the manifestation. "He smiled, but I didn't trust him." "She's such a phony!" Successful liars are some of the best shape-shifters around, posing as friends, confidants, demure innocents, or solicitous caregivers. Everyone in the audience at a performance of *Othello* has to wonder how anyone could trust the slimy flattery of the villian Iago. How could Othello have bought into that treachery? Of course we know that Shakespeare's character ignored the signs of Iago's body language and believed what he wanted to believe. Perhaps Othello suffered from brain damage to the part of the amygdala that helps the brain recognize menacing or dangerous faces. We, too, delude ourselves regularly—in our relationships ("But you said you loved me!")

and at work ("I've got everything under control"), and we lie to others almost as a matter of course.

I always have to laugh when I run into a student in the hallway who has just skipped my class and she sighs, saying, "Oh, I'm sorry, I was soooo sick this morning, I just couldn't make it." At the same time they think it's inappropriate to say, "Sorry teach, I decided to blow you off this morning to have a fight with my boyfriend, or to sleep late, or to get a haircut. . . ." They sigh deeply, tilt their heads, roll their eyes up to the left, and shrug. I silently wish them better luck at lying when they go out into the world and take the day off from work! A student of mine recently sent me a card with an illustration of a man speaking at a function. The caption read "You can tell a politician is lying when he is moving his lips."

Deception is a successful survival strategy in the animal world—from the uncanny mimicry in certain orchids, designed to lure unsuspecting pollinators, to the simple strategies of a mother bird flying away from her nest in order to trick a predator into thinking that her home is elsewhere. Animals play dead or pretend to be wounded in order to survive. You can't win a poker game if you don't have a command of both your body language and that of your opponents.

How do you recognize a lie? We often ignore the signals liars send: "He seemed like such a nice guy!" "Who would have thought she was capable of that?" Con men throughout history have relied on people's willingness to deceive themselves when it comes to money.

This question doesn't just apply to our relationships with others. Since we know by now that our gestures and posture are a reflection of our own emotions, your body language can also reveal to you how you lie to yourself. David McNeill, author of *The Face, A Natural History,* suggests that certain ways of lying to yourself are also a kind of survival strategy: "Litigators know they can argue a case more effectively if they persuade themselves the client is right, and salespeople routinely pump themselves up about the product." In a society based on competition, what's important is to win, not necessarily to be honest. This intentional self-deception is useful. But what about our habitual rationalizations, excuses for failures, and outbursts of defensive righteous indignation where we convince ourselves to live a lie?

Jim is an attractive, successful man who had a severe accident and had taken a year off from his high-profile career to heal. He was torn among three directions: an excellent job offer in his old field, the possibility of starting a new business, and chucking it all to spend a year writing a book. As we talked, Jim quickly eliminated the job offer. He himself noticed that each time he talked about the recently concluded phone interview he held his breath and clenched his teeth. As he spoke with enthusiasm about launching his new prod-uct, his shoulders rounded, then moved alternately forward—as if he was shouldering his way through a crowd. His hands kept pushing forward as he spoke: "This product will go, I know it. I just have to push ahead now." Then he spoke about the book. As he spoke about walks on the beach, getting his thoughts onto paper, his shoulders dropped and he took a deep breath. His right hand became graceful as it arched through the air, often gently touching his breastbone before floating outward again. He went back and forth several times between options—it was like watching two people trying to take possession of the same body. I asked him if he felt any different when talking about the two subjects. He had not. I then mirrored his body language for each. After he finished laughing at the obvious message he was sending himself, he confessed that throughout his career he had always done what he should do in order to be successful. He agreed that it might be time to try something that made his heart sing.

The key element in Jim's story is that he himself did not see his body language until it was pointed out to him. We are so good at creating blinds to protect ourselves that it can be almost impossible to catch the truth. Observing others can be just as difficult. Of-ten it's just a fleeting movement of the eyes or a slight raise of the shoulder that betrays the inner truth of a person's words.

Paul Ekman, who made the study of the face his life's work, developed the Facial Action Coding System, a complex method for analyzing the muscles in the face and the expressions of the face. Ekman codified and classified all the muscles in the face and the different expressions we are capable of. The Facial Action Coding System is currently used by groups as varied as sales forces and military intelligence. Ekman gives as an example the story of Mary, a suicidal woman who was interviewed by the hospital and then released for a weekend leave. As Mary was checking out of the hospital, she confessed to the doctor that she just wanted to go home so she could kill herself. The shocked doctors didn't understand how they could have misread her interview—she had seemed so much better. Ekman was called in to analyze the film of Mary's interview to help them learn how to determine when suicidal patients were lying. They "played it over and over for dozens of hours, examining in slow motion every gesture and expression. Finally they saw it. As Mary's doctor asked her about her plans for the future, a look of utter despair flashed across her face so quickly that it was almost imperceptible."

FACING THE TRUTH

Many times we sabotage our true intentions with unnecessary actions—for example, cleaning the entire house in order not to make a crucial phone call. Or we try to do something that we truly don't want—settling for a boring job, perhaps—and succeed at neither.

Don sat despondently near my desk. "Did you get the job?" *I asked.*

"No." *He shook his head.* "As the guy was describing the responsibilities, I could feel myself tensing, thinking to myself,* What am I thinking? I'm an artist, not a manager! *I don't want to sit there creating spec ads for some stupid tire company, or worse!* But I really need the money, so I'm sitting there in the office, nodding my head as he's talking about staff meetings, strategies for clients. After he lays it all out to me, he says, 'So do you think you can handle this kind of role?' 'Sure,' I say. I feel like my shoulders are up around my ears. My hand keeps rubbing my nose. The tension in my eyes feels like* *my brain is about to explode. When we shake hands, I grip him so hard he winces. The one thing I got out of that interview is the confirmation that I definitely don't want to work in advertising!"*

People often wish to be able to catch liars by telltale signals, like Don's nose rubbing or the eye rolling above, but often the lie is the incongruence between two gestures. Mary's fleeting expression of despair was incongruent with her words, but we focus so much on words that we often miss the revelatory moment. There is a saying: "Language was created so that men could lie." Becoming aware of your own incongruent gestures can help you recognize the lies you are living. In the book's opening I asked the question "Are you who you say are?" Why don't things go as planned? Why can't you achieve your fondest wishes and desires? It is this unconscious self-deception that is often at the root of your failures. All of this is reflected in your carriage. Unfortunately these are the habitual postures that are so ingrained that they take a lot of practice to recognize. And often even when we say we *want* to see them and to change, the truth is that change can be absolutely terrifying. How can you admit to yourself that the reason you never quit the job at the insurance agency is really because you think you are a terrible writer and will waste your time trying to write that screenplay? How can you possibly find a man who respects you when you keep pushing nice men away or running from them? All this can be seen in your body language—if you are willing to look.

Jonathon took a course with me, stating up front that what he wanted was to find a meaningful sexual relationship. He was unable to understand why every woman he met treated him like a pal, a confidant, but was never physically interested. Jonathon's need was urgent—he wanted to raise a family and it was clear he'd make a wonderful father. Jonathon is a reasonably attractive, extremely intelligent, and sensitive man with a great capacity for love. What was the problem? One day I watched him in the dining room outside of class. Each time an attractive woman he knew came by his shoulders raised up and came forward as the back of his head sank down, curving his neck. He smiled as he looked up, creating the impression of a shy eight-year-old looking up, expectantly waiting for a pat or kiss on the head. "Hi Sheila, hee hee," he'd say, the "hee hee" being almost like a tic, his shoulders jerking a little forward as this inadvertent hiccup of an expression came out. No wonder women didn't look at him as a sex object!

As we continued to work together, Jonathon began to unravel the stories behind his postural choices. By the end of the semester he was able to separate his shoulders from his head and even occasionally look a woman directly in the eye.

FOLLOWING THE YES

Many times people will recognize that their body language belies their stated intention. This book introduces you to people who have made discoveries about their carriages, their habits, and presentation that interfere with their stated goals. Sometimes it is useful to change one's posture intentionally. But sometimes, no matter how hard you try, you can't seem to change it. Traditionally we are taught to force the issue: Stand up straight! Give a strong handshake! Look him in the eye! But it reads as false, because it is forced.

Our culture puts an emphasis on pushing past resistance, without understanding the source or the learning that resistance can provide. Immersion therapy, intense workouts, and sayings like "Push through the pain" are some ways we try to compel change. I propose exploring another way, going where it is easy, where you already have permission— call it following the yes. Instead of fighting a habit, support it.

Some people might say, "Well, isn't that just giving up? Just going downstream?" But it's not as simple as that, because at every moment you are given a choice. You can automatically continue in the same grooves you have behaved in for your whole life. Or you can try to counter and fight your habits by forcing yourself to do the opposite— engaging even more tension and compulsive behavior. Or you can look at each moment as an invitation and listen to whether there is a yes in you, and pay attention to that. For example, when Jonathon noticed how his shoulder hunching belied his intention to flirt, instead of trying to force his shoulders to stay down he explored his shoulders, slowly following their natural pattern, and inviting them to go even higher! Then, once he knew everything about the pattern his shoulders were taking, he invited them to move in other ways. Often they would not move. And sometimes, to his surprise, he'd notice that he was also holding his breath or clenching his teeth. Each time this happened he would look for ways to make it safe to say yes to something before moving.

This practice can be done both at home and out in the world. You can experiment with the exercise at home either lying or sitting down. Choose a movement—perhaps it's the raising of the shoulders. Or perhaps it's rounding the back. Begin to attend to what you do—how far do you go easily? Where is the constriction? What are your emotions, if any, as you move? When you get to the "no," don't push. Instead, go back to where the yes is clear and explore in another direction. Or approach your stopping point from another angle. Like unknotting a tangled thread, you go back to where things move freely. You will find that this small experiment will change the way you carry yourself when you go out.

When you are out—in a work or social situation—you can do the same thing, although it can be more challenging. For example, you are out shopping on a day when you called in sick, your baseball cap covering not just your unwashed hair but shading your un-made-up eyes, and suddenly, out of the corner of your eye, you see your boss. You could quickly duck around to another aisle and hope he didn't recognize you. You could torture yourself by waiting till he looks up and try to figure out what to say. Or you could take a moment to notice what is happening to your breathing, your posture. Is this familiar? Is this some kind of fear? You may find that suddenly you realize it's okay to tell the truth. "Hey, sorry I couldn't come in today, I was feeling pretty sick and I needed to get some chamomile tea. I hope to be better tomorrow." Or maybe not. It just may be too much this time. If you do go around the corner, follow your breath. Know that you are not escaping from him—you are learning something about yourself. The important thing in following the yes is to first ask the questions—is it okay to go here? How do I feel? If you never ask, you will always run, or repeat the same gestures, or say the same thing.

Once you begin to acknowledge the yes and the no in yourself, you will begin to catch the lies you tell yourself more easily. And as you recognize this in yourself, you will start to see these same movements in others.

WATCHING MY WALK

P. D. Ouspensky, an early twentieth-century philosopher, once offered the following equation: "Effort plus motive equals result." Moshe Feldenkrais, who will be introduced in more depth in Chapter 3, offered a similar one: "Less effort plus more attention yields a greater result." If you can keep these two maxims in mind as you aim for your goals, you will begin to see clearly what gets in the way of your stated aim. If, for example, you say you want to be an award-winning writer, but your motives are based on desperately needing public validation, then many of your efforts will be strained, your point of view in your writing will be affected by your need for approval. In this case you are living a lie because your motive is not what you say it is. Even if you do sell your screenplay, it will never feel like enough. If, on the other hand, you begin with the same aim but pay attention to your attitude and efforts while constantly clarifying your motives and approaches, you may find that you no longer need validation to do your work. Your work will improve and you will succeed. Or you may discover that this ambition is something you've carried from childhood to please your parents, and that you really want to be a gardener, and this now pleases you. If you have the right motive but your efforts are scattered, compulsive, or self-sabotaging, you still will never get what you want. Your efforts then belie your motive. Only by attending to your impulses will you be able to see what is really necessary to achieve satisfaction. It may be shocking and frustrating at times, but the rewards can be immeasurable.

Mark came to my group classes after a lifetime of athletic performance that had left him with pain in many areas—particularly the back, shoulders, and neck. Each time I would give instructions to the class, Mark would reach farther than anyone in the class, stretch his leg higher, roll faster. After class he would complain that everything still hurt. I would suggest to him that he try doing less movement, move more slowly, and listen to what is interfering. Each time he would nod, then get back on the floor and hurt himself again. For Mark everything was about performance. Only more, bigger, stronger counted. This kept him from seeing how he was actually hurting himself in the process. He approached each movement in his habitual way, looking clumsy in the bargain, since he didn't really attend to how *he did anything.*

THE TRUTH SHALL SET YOU FREE

In order to get the most out of this work, it's useful to state some goals and have a systematic process of tracking your development. You can do this any way you want: journaling, creating art projects, making a chart. I have included a worksheet on page 172 that you may find helpful. You can copy the categories on separate sheets of paper, photocopy the layout from the book, or you can download the form from my Web site: www.laviniaplonka.com.

I have also included a sample goal to give you some ideas. You will notice that these worksheets break both your effort and motive into three parts: physical, mental, and emotional. These may not be easy to differentiate right now, but throughout the book we will explore these three ways of studying yourself. If something doesn't seem clear for now, leave it blank or just write down your immediate response. You are learning a new way of seeing, and until you have more practice you will experience blind spots in yourself. As you continue this study, both your motives and efforts will become clearer.

I recommend that you use a separate worksheet for each goal. Track your progress by filling sheets out periodically. Once a week is ideal. You will discover that what you see and *how* you see changes as you move through the book.

This is difficult work, and uncovering the lies we tell ourselves is a subject rich enough for an entire book. But beginning this process from the point of view of your body language is an opening toward greater self-knowledge—and with the right attitude it can even be fun.

Exploration Checklist

- ☐ Practice following the yes.
- ☐ Create Goal/Motive/Effort worksheets.

Three

IS IT SCIENCE OR MAGIC?

Nothing is so unfamiliar to man as himself.

François Delsarte

*P*ut your palm on your upper chest. Stay there a minute. Do you suddenly feel the need to recite the Pledge of Allegiance? Or perhaps to recite a few lines of poetry to your loved one? Now put your palm on your solar plexus area (just below the rib cage in the center of your body). Different, right? Just try saying the Pledge of Allegiance with your hand down there. Why? Is it just cultural? It seems not. Certain gestures and expressions are the same all over the world.

Knowledge of the power of body language can be traced back to ancient times. The Natyasastra, a Sanskrit text probably written around 200 CE but possibly centuries older contains verse upon verse of body language analysis. In the Greek and Roman empires the study of gesture and body language was taught to actors, poets, and politicians. Even Augustus Caesar studied how to use gesture along with his oratory. Certain hand movements evoke powerful responses around the world—from the mudras of India to the sacred gestures of Catholic and Orthodox priests.

Artists and actors depict characters that evoke emotions in us through how they draw the character. What makes us recognize the Shakespearean villain Iago on stage before he utters a word? When you approach a painting in a museum, how is it that even from a distance, even without a halo, you know it is a picture of a holy person? There is a language hidden in plain sight that we all intuitively understand yet pretend doesn't exist. Why?

Our language is filled with metaphors related to the body. "Her heart fell." "He became weak in the knees." "You're always sticking your nose into other people's business." These metaphors speak volumes on the correspondences among our carriage, emotional state, and health. Yet it is only recently that science has begun to study these relationships.

Psychoneuroimmunology and neurocardiology are only two of the newer fields of medicine that are looking at systemic connections throughout the human organism. Neurocardiology posits that the heart is actually another brain, an emotional brain. There are direct neurological links between the heart and the head brain. Ideas like emotional intelligence begin to have new resonance in the light of this research. Suddenly "I know it in my heart," "Follow your heart," and so on, have a deeper meaning. Heart disease is just one aspect of the body language mystery that neurocardiology is exploring. Psychoneuroimmunology concerns itself with relationships within the entire body-mind system. Researchers are looking at the body as a network instead of separately functioning parts. As the term implies, psychoneuroimmunology studies the effects of the mind on the immune system and vice versa, perhaps explaining why certain alternative health approaches are so effective. From iridology (diagnosing the body by studying the iris of the eye) to acupuncture (part of Chinese medicine), holistic medicine looks at the body "holographically," each part reflecting the whole, the emotions affecting the physiology, the carriage affecting the emotions, and so on. This holographic principle has been part of the art of healing at least as far back as ancient Egypt.

The relation of posture to emotional experience has also been observed and catalogued. Paul Ekman observed that when you spend a certain amount of time with a particular facial expression you begin to actually feel the emotion. Susana Bloch, a Chilean neuroscientist, has also done significant research into physical expression, codifying not just facial expression but posture and respiratory patterns. In her early research working with hypnosis, she placed her subjects in the postures and respiratory patterns of various emotions. Soon these hypnotized subjects began to experience the emotion they had been placed in. She found this process of taking on the posture so effective that she developed an acting technique based on her research called the Alba Emoting Method, which is currently taught around the world. This method is designed to help actors "step in and step out" of emotional states without needing to draw on personal memories by understanding the relationship between the body and emotions.

Ekman and Bloch theorize that all of our emotional expressions come from six basic or primal reactions. However, their categories do not exactly correspond.

EKMAN	BLOCH
Disgust	Tenderness
Anger	Anger
Fear	Fear
Happiness	Joy
Sadness	Sadness
Surprise	Eroticism/Lust

Ekman believes that lust, like pain, is not an emotion because it can (according to him) be felt in specific parts of the body, whereas he feels that emotions like anger cannot be pinpointed. Bloch, on the other hand, believes that emotions like disgust and surprise are actually mixed emotions. The Natyasastra, mentioned above, lists eight basic emotions, including disgust, surprise, and "amorousness," which it differentiates from "eroticness." Interestingly, joy or happiness is not included in the basic emotions, but laughter is. In many ways contemporary research is rediscovering what has been hidden in plain sight for centuries.

While we like to think that our expression of emotions is what differentiates us from animals, the fact is that all of the above emotions can be observed in animal behavior. Much has been written about the animal roots of some of our body language. Charles Darwin, the father of evolutionary theory, recorded his observations in a book, *The Expression of the Emotions in Man and Animals.* Zoologist and ethologist Desmond Morris's many books and TV series, from *The Naked Ape* to *The Human Animal,* have demonstrated that our smiles, frowns, and stamping feet are all primal survival strategies. The remarkable correspondence between what we call emotion and animal behavior can be disconcerting. It suggests that perhaps very little of what we do is really intentional, but merely a reaction that connects us to our primitive forbears. However, studying this connection can help us to better understand the forces that cause our heads and hearts to sink, why we strut when proud and pleased, and how to use these very reactions to begin to live an embodied life.

These primal emotions, and the mixed emotional reactions, such as envy, shame, and pride, are triggered by stimuli in our environment, but they are not "where we live." Throughout most of the course of the day we think we are in neutral: walking down the street, driving, sitting at the computer, doing laundry. An emotional reaction can be triggered—a moment of road rage, noticing that your jeans got bleached, running into an admirer. But what goes on in between reactions? Neurologist Antonio Damasio suggests that there are what he calls "background emotions" constantly informing your state. These are what color your emotional reactions. For example, if you are in a funk, bad news will make you feel worse, and you may just sigh when you hear good news. Ekman, on the other hand, does not qualify these states as emotions, instead calling them moods. Whatever you choose to call these states, they have an impact on the people you meet and how you go about getting what you want (and don't want!) from life. These background emotions or moods are much more difficult to recognize because they are what form your perceptions of reality. It's like trying to look at your face without a mirror. While we will examine how to recognize emotions, we will also study these subtler manifestations as well.

Have an Emotional Day!

Carry a notebook or piece of paper around for a day. Each time you find yourself experiencing an emotion, jot it down. At the end of the day, add them up—how many times were you angry? Frustrated? Happy? Or did you not notice any emotions at all?

INTRODUCING THE TOOLS

Delsarte's System of Expression

In the early nineteenth century François Delsarte ruined his voice at a bad elocution school. He then became determined to understand the science behind effective oratory. His research revealed that gesture and body language were powerful aspects of communication. He once said, "Gesture is the lightning, words are the thunder." Contemporary science has revealed that our unconscious gestures precede our spoken thoughts and that often, it is these very gestures that betray us. Delsarte studied ancient history, went to morgues, spent countless hours observing people, and experimented on himself and his students. His elegant system presents the human body as a network based on a trinity of functions: mental, physical, and emotional. He claimed his understanding came from studying ancient art. His observations anticipated much of modern biology's discoveries regarding brain function and the nervous system.

By studying human behavior, he was able to intuit information that has been borne out by modern medicine and scientists like Ekman. For example, you can see in the

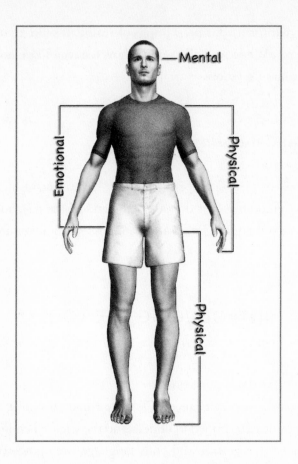

illustration that Delsarte classifed the head as the mental zone, an obvious choice. He also subdivided it into zones. He called the front of the skull the mental zone, the center the emotional zone, and the back of the skull the vital or physical zone. We now know that while operating as a whole, the brain does seem to have certain functions that relate to Delsarte's divisions: the neocortex governing our logical reasoning functions, the central or limbic brain governing the secretion of hormones that influence our emotional life, and the parietal brain/sensory cortex, which regulates our nervous system and motor functions.

Delsarte was not operating from the contemporary scientist's perspective. His system was entirely based on personal experience and observation. His work is not presented here as science but as an invitation for you to experiment and verify the experience for yourself. When training actors and orators, Delsarte repeatedly cautioned that the gesture meant nothing if the actor was not trying to sense himself at the same time, in order to understand and to *embody* the emotion contained in the gesture.

Delsarte also included divisions of the eyes, eyebrows, hands, fingers, mouth, and so on, continuing to delineate smaller and smaller fractions of the self, not unlike a fractal. But he stressed that everything should be viewed in relation to the whole.

Predating Susana Bloch's experiments by 150 years, he also spoke of how taking a posture can evoke the experience of an emotion. He cites an example of a soldier being put into the posture of fear under hypnosis, then shortly afterward manifesting all the symptoms of terror. He cautioned, however, that one should consider the suggestibility of the subject, the intent of the experimenter, and one's belief in the outcome. In that way he anticipated some current debates on scientists' attitudes and their influence on the results of their experiments. Still, there is more than sufficient evidence of a correlation among posture, attitude, and emotion, even taking all these factors into consideration. Dr. Bloch's hypnosis experiments have removed some of these subjective roadblocks, but not all.

Delsarte suggested that the ancient Greeks used this knowledge in the creation of their art in order to evoke specific responses in the viewer, not unlike the ideas presented in the Natyasastra.

Body and Mature Behavior

In the 1940s Dr. Moshe Feldenkrais was known in Europe as a scientist (working with the Curies) and as an athlete. He was one of the first European black belts in judo, and he was instrumental in bringing the Japanese martial arts to the West. By accident he found himself literally brought to his knees: two crippling injuries left him virtually unable to walk.

Feldenkrais plunged himself into research, using himself as the laboratory, in hopes of recovering his lost mobility. Infant development, brain function, movement patterns, and animal motor behavior were some of the areas he studied in his quest for understanding movement. The result is a sophisticated yet simple system for teaching people how to observe their habitual movement patterns and develop new choices in movement, thus improving physical, mental, and emotional quality of life.

The Feldenkrais Method of Somatic Education teaches awareness through movement. Feldenkrais observed that at every moment four things are going on—thinking, feeling (emotion), sensing, and movement. Even when we are still, we are moving via the breath and the autonomic functions. Even when we are playing, we are thinking—the mind is present, taking in information, responding to each situation. And as mentioned earlier, even when we think we are neutral, background emotions that we are barely aware of are present. If you did not notice any emotions during your day, it really just means you were not aware of them—they are always there!

Throughout the book there are exercises and experiments to try based on those developed by Dr. Feldenkrais. Unlike traditional exercises, these sequences are most effective when done with a minimum of physical effort. If you slow down and do minimal movement, you are able to sense more about your patterns than if you do large, strenuous movements. The challenge becomes not "how well can I do these movements?" but "how much do I notice as I do these movements?" When performing any movement sequence ask yourself the following questions: "Am I comfortable?" "Am I interested?" "Am I paying attention?" Feldenkrais believed that learning should be a pleasurable experience. He once said, "If you're not having fun, you're not learning." Remember to keep this open, playful approach to your study, and you will benefit far more than if you take it on as a chore.

THE THEATER OF LIFE

The theater traditionally has been the mirror of our behavior—our passions, foibles, foolishness, and sorrows. An actor is trained to use his body to evoke the experience of a character so that when we see him on the stage there is the shock of recognition that reminds us of our own connections to these experiences. As I said earlier, every person I meet is a story unfolding. The walk, the stance, the facial expressions all tell me the history, the longings, the fears of an individual. There are as many ways to train an actor as there are styles of music or art. Each style offers another avenue for self study. This book features explorations that come from the more technical aspects of an actor's training—the kind of work we call "from the outside in." Instead of trying to evoke memories or emotions and then examining how they affect our posture, we will explore techniques for "stepping into" another's shoes in order to understand how to inhabit more fully our own. These exercises come from a number of sources other than Delsarte and Feldenkrais: the work of theater innovators Jerzy Grotowski and Peter Brook, mime exercises from both the French and Polish tradition, commedia dell'arte, and Indian acting. By playing with an actor's vocabulary you will quicken your own ability to sense what you and others are saying behind mere words. You will see that indeed "All the world's a stage, and all the men and women merely players." After reading this book, you will be better able to choose your role, and perhaps even choose the play you are in.

Exploration Checklist

- ☐ Explore the emotions of your day.
- ☐ Set aside a time each day and create a space at home for exploring movement.

Part Two

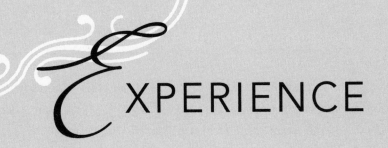

EXPERIENCE

*T*here is no experience in any part of you that does not resonate throughout the whole rest of yourself. You can't simply isolate a shoulder or a vertebra and understand what is taking place. By the same token, each part contains within it information about the whole self. The position of your knees can tell a lot about what your back is doing; how you carry your head can tell everything from your sense of safety to the fact that you have to wear orthotics in your shoes. This section will examine the parts of the self, but remember always to consider your explorations from the point of view of the whole.

Four

A LEG TO STAND ON

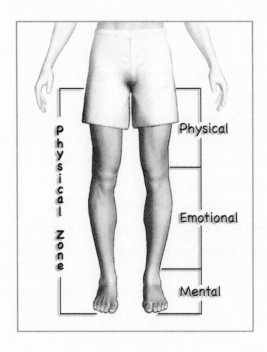

My legs carry me where I want to go.
    Where do I want to go?
My legs support me in my work. What is
    my work?

STANDING YOUR GROUND

Why do some people have flat feet? Does locking your knees back say something to others? What is a position of strength? How you stand affects every part of your personal organization, and inversely all aspects of your carriage are reflected in your stance. If your feet roll in, or your toes point out to the sides, or your heels don't touch the ground, your back, your hips, everything is affected, as is how people perceive you.

Your legs literally are your support system. They hold up the rest of you, not an easy or practical feat from a design perspective. Being on all fours is much more stable and distributes weight more evenly. To balance one hundred to three hundred pounds standing upward of six feet into the air on two small points requires extremely good organization, or else either tension occurs or we fall over. Since most of us don't spend our day falling over, nor are we organized in perfect neutral equilibrium, we can assume that there are some tensions in any chosen stance. Do you stand with legs wide apart, like a soldier at rest? Perhaps the weight is all on one leg, the other leg bent and pointing slightly outward. Where are your feet? If someone were to come from behind and gently push your knees, would they collapse? Move softly forward? Hold tightly?

Delsarte placed the legs in what he called the physical zone. From his point of view, not only do the legs hold you up, but they, along with the arms, are the workhorses of the body. They help you push, lift, climb, run—in other words, they get the job done. When we say someone doesn't have a leg to stand on, we mean that the person has no foundation for his argument. To stand your ground, stand up for yourself, not take something sitting down, are all sayings that reflect the vitality and power in the legs. The nature of your stance can tell a lot about you and your reactions to a situation. Delsarte's trinity division continues: the thighs are the physical part of the physical zone, the calves/shins are the emotional part, and the feet are the mental part. The first can be understood simply. Think of the thighs as the powerhouse, the support system of the leg (and body). They do the physical work.

It's hard at first to imagine that any part of the leg would express emotions. And yet there is an emotional component to how we use our legs. Delsarte believed that our emotions are connected with where our attention is. When walking, the lower legs extend forward and your attention and interest is on where you are going. When standing they are directly underneath you, neutral. If, however, while standing you bend your knee, crossing one calf over the other, you are bringing your attention into yourself. Think of a Don Juan type, leaning against a building, legs crossed, waiting for a pretty girl. Or a moment when someone is criticizing you and you shift your weight to one leg, bringing the other knee in, slightly bent. Even the quality of the lower leg reflects aspects of emotional life. While someone with bulging thigh muscles presents a picture of strength, someone with bulging calf muscles presents a picture of tension. Overdeveloped calf muscles indicate a struggle for stability, rigidity in one's walk, perhaps some kind of compulsiveness—workaholism, addiction to exercise. Bulging calves affect the feet and the hips, and vice versa. Skinny, undeveloped calves, on the other hand, lend an air of immaturity, flightiness. As a matter of fact, in ages past one way character was judged was by the shape of the calf. Back when men wore tights their calves revealed their nobility, their stature in life. Men even used padding to give dimension to skinny, flabby calves.

The feet are the mental part. They go where your mind is—one foot in front of the other, stopping on a dime. A tapping foot is an impatient mind. You can trip over your own feet when your mind is wandering!

As Feldenkrais noted, a static posture is uncomfortable. We rarely stand in one position for any length of time. But you still can learn a lot about someone by their stance as well as their walk.

The following illustrations are the basis of the myriad positions we take in standing. There are perhaps hundreds of variations when you take into account position of feet, other aspects of asymmetrical standing, and one-legged poses. Delsarte had specific classifications for each position with a complicated nomenclature. For simplicity's sake, in each section I will focus on basic postures and their relationship to the plumb line.

NOTE ON OBSERVING

Delsarte noted that our physical postures could indicate "a condition or a sentiment," and he stressed the importance of looking at the whole picture. A condition is a bodily state—such as exhaustion, injury, drunkenness. A sentiment is an emotional state—

such as arrogance, love, jealousy. When you observe someone it is important to recognize the difference between the two! Standing in a crowded elevator with your legs glued together and your arms smashed by your sides expresses something completely different than standing that way at a cocktail party. Arms crossed around the chest while standing in sub-zero temperature is not a sentiment; it's just an attempt to be warm. Always consider the situation as well as the person.

Attitudes of the Legs

Try each of these postures for yourself and see how they make you feel.

NOTE: Where you place your toes in relation to your heels creates another nine possibilities in standing, which create nuances in our characters as well. The following positions keep the foot along the same trajectory as the leg, but, feel free to experiment.

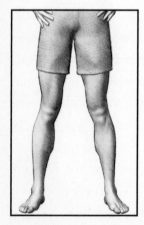

1. Legs are hip or shoulder width apart.

It is interesting that the military has adopted this posture as "parade rest" as opposed to "attention." Many people choose this position, thinking that it is one of strength and manliness, like the Jolly Green Giant. But in actual fact it is a very unstable and inflexible position, especially if you separate the legs to shoulder width. If someone were to push you from either the front or behind, it would be easy to fall. The straight knees make it difficult to move to the sides or to turn around. Standing like this can mean overconfidence or trying to give the impression that you are the man of the house. This posture can indicate conditions such as fatigue, vertigo, and intoxication. Emotional states (sentiments) range from feeling comfortable and familiar to macho braggadocio.

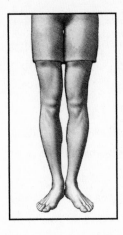

2. Both legs are together, knees straight, heels together, weight centered.

Delsarte called this the "position of the inferior before the superior." A child listening to an elder, a soldier before a superior officer, a person who feels smaller than the person they are listening to will assume this posture. This person does not have a lot of movement options and is in a weakened position.

3. Place the heel of one foot at the instep of the other so that they are at right angles. Then bring that foot away in a straight line. Stand centered between the two feet.

This is a transition pose. You could go in any direction from here. Therefore it can indicate anything from a fighter getting ready for action (this is a common martial arts stance—look at any Bruce Lee movie) to someone caught in indecision—"Which way should I go?"

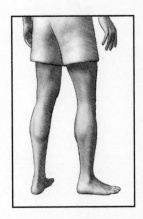

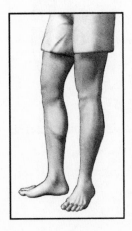

4. Put your weight on the back leg, which is straight. The forward leg is a little to the side, slightly bent, with not much weight on it.

This is a receptive, sometimes thinking position. Delsarte called it the attitude of a thinker or scholar. When your weight is on the back leg in this way you are not going anywhere. It means you are engaged in what's happening either internally or in your conversation. You have an attitude toward the other person. You can feel how this attitude shifts simply by changing the weight from the back foot, or sinking deeper into your standing hip, or moving your front foot. You'll see that your way of listening—from objectivity to derisive judgment—changes.

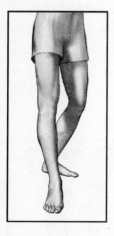

5. Once again, the weight is on the back leg, but this time that back leg is bent. The front leg is extended somewhere to the front or slightly side with the leg straight.

When you take this position, feel what the upper part of the self has to do to maintain equilibrium. You are retreating so you must bend forward. It's a position that relates to submission, depression, even sorrow. An exaggerated version of this posture is the way courtly men bowed to ladies. We take this position when giving in, surrendering, offering.

6. The weight is once again on the straight back leg, and the front leg is straight and forward.

Most of us avoid this kind of confrontational posture. Delsarte noted that sometimes people mistake this posture as a "manly pose," when the effect is often the opposite. In commedia dell'arte, the Italian comedy of the Renaissance, this would have been a position for El Capitano—a bragging fool. Imagine Mandy Patinkin in *Princess Bride,* or Errol Flynn in any movie, and you have this pose—somewhere between the hero and the fool.

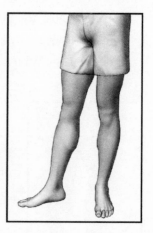

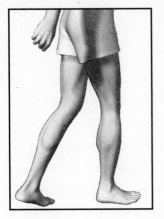

7. This time the weight is forward, the back leg is behind, knee slightly bent, heel off the ground.

This is an action pose—you are definitely going forward.

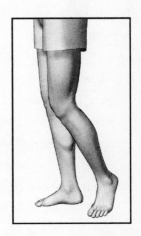

8. Weight is on the front leg, the back leg only slightly behind—as if you just took a step.

Changing direction, changing your mind, shifting gears, pausing in mid-thought are all reflected in this position.

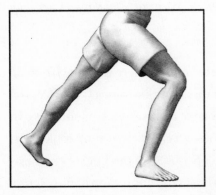

9. Weight is on a bent front leg, back leg is extended, heel up.

Wahoo! Don't get in the way of someone like this. This is an action posture—one that is rarely held. Think of grabbing a child from the edge of a cliff or earnestly entreating the woman you love.

ON BENDED KNEE

The expressions "I was brought to my knees" and "My knees went weak" literally are true. Collapsing knees is a neurochemical response that has been observed in patients with narcolepsy, cataplexy, and various diseases such as multiple sclerosis where the legs suddenly give out. How is this connected with our emotional experience? Moments of grief and despair often literally bring us to our knees. "I just can't stand it anymore" can manifest in knee problems, from tendonitis to arthritis. Shock, grief, and awe all invite system collapse. Is this connected with why we kneel when we pray? Why people knelt before the king? An acknowledgment of our own weakness in the face of something greater?

Marlene came to me with a chronic knee problem. "When did this begin?" I asked her. She gave a wry smile. "I literally tripped over myself," she replied. As we worked together, a story emerged of the last five years attending her dying father. She was the youngest child and was extremely attached to her father. Even though Marlene is well educated and talented, she has relied on Dad for financial and emotional support, never able to maintain a real career or any long-term romantic relationship. When he died she was devastated, really unable to see how she could continue. "Tripping over herself" was the final straw for her already destabilized system, and her knee gave out. Although Marlene is working to recover her stability, her attachment to her father and her fear of "standing on her own two feet" continues to keep her in pain.

When knees don't line up with the bones of the legs and feet there is undue strain on the joints. Something else has to compensate—back muscles, ankle muscles. The feet roll in, often creating flat feet. The impression created is one of awkwardness, clumsiness. In fact, it is difficult to move powerfully with this kind of stance. Quick turning could twist the knee. Running will jar and compromise the joint. A person with this kind of organization of the knees will be careful, tentative, which reinforces the impression of impotence.

PUTTING YOUR BEST FOOT FORWARD

Sometimes feet get ruined by shoes—pointy high heels, tight ice skates, ballet pointe shoes are just a few culprits. A colleague of mine teaches a workshop entitled "Surviving Pumps." Our shoe choices reflect aspects of our personalities as well—the personality that chooses sensible shoes versus the personality that resonates with Carrie Bradshaw's Manolo Blahniks. But many foot problems are connected to how the foot is used in standing and walking. Bunions, hammer toes, and corns often reflect the nature of the stance. For example, many people have no idea that they stand with their toes curling in their shoes. Besides creating foot problems, this communicates a sense of rigidity and tension (it's hard to change direction easily if your toes are stuck). Bunions are often the result of a slight rolling in (pronation) of the foot over many years. This rolling has many causes—from tension in the back and hips to compensating for where the knee or the foot is pointing. It is very difficult to walk assertively if your feet point outward. And at the same time it's not just about changing where your feet are.

Nathan came to me with shoulder injuries. He was a bulky, jolly sort, with a huge barrel chest, a loud and easy laugh, and a kind of waddling walk. As I observed his walk it was clear to me that one of the reasons he had injured his shoulders was that his torso was one solid mass, so that there was no movement in the shoulder girdle. There was something very forced about how he put one leg in front of another. After our lesson, Nathan was alarmed that even though his shoulder pain was relieved as he walked, his feet pointed outward slightly. "I've worked so hard to get my feet to go straight," he exclaimed. Apparently Nathan had suffered much ridicule as a teen for his "duck walk." He had forced his feet to turn inward without understanding how that might affect all the other parts of his organization that contribute to his pattern. This created a tense double bind in his walking pattern that caused everything to become more or less frozen, resulting in many injuries, the latest of which was the shoulders. By working with all of Nathan's habits, we began to unwind the patterns that originally had created the feet pointing out. It turns out that

Nathan's jolly, goofy demeanor was congruent with his pointy-toed, side-to-side waddle. As his feet straightened out, his chest softened and his walk became more fluid, and Nathan was able to develop a smoother, more mature approach to people, relationships, and the choices he made. In addition, he has begun to "seriously" pursue a career in humor.

(LITERALLY) WALKING YOUR TALK

The U.S. government has revealed a satellite surveillance device that can identify a person from his walk. Although only 80 percent effective at the moment, technology is rapidly improving to enable us to actually fingerprint the gait. As mentioned in Chapter 2, even when you think you are neutral your walk is giving you away.

Walking has been described as falling and catching yourself, over and over. Each time you take a step a trajectory of force is moving from your foot to your head. How that force is conducted, where it jams up, and how the rest of the skeleton moves in response are just some of the ways your walk indicates personality.

William is not a big guy. But you wouldn't know it from the sound of his walk. Every step he takes reverberates throughout the building. His heels smack down onto the floor with so much power that your chair shakes. If you were walking down the street and you saw William barreling down, you'd jump out of the way so you wouldn't get plowed down. Thing is, William is a really nice guy. And he wants people to like him. But his bearing is so forceful that he often puts people off or intimidates them. Not only that, but his back is really sore. How are these challenges related to the way William walks?

William's story is a rich one. His walk is the result of many factors—from an unconscious imitation of his forceful father to his own perceived need to seem larger in order to be noticed. He was picked on in school for his size, and he joined the wrestling team in order to become stronger. Instead of shrinking or retreating into purely intellectual pursuits, William pushed, stormed, and stomped his way to being noticed. As he grew older, these strategies became habits. Even when William no longer needed to defend himself, his walk created a barrier between himself and the people he wanted to meet.

Learning to read a walk can be a book in itself, because walking is a full-body activity. Throughout the book I will refer back to the walk as we examine the impact of our other parts on this daily activity. For now we can examine how the way we use of our feet and legs affects our walk.

THE MECHANICS OF WALKING ☽

As mentioned earlier, Feldenkrais believed that learning should be a pleasurable experience—so as you try this and later movement explorations, make sure that you are comfortable. Only do as much movement as is easy. If a movement is painful or difficult, look at your options. You can do less. You can find a different way to do the movement that is more comfortable for you. Or you can just rest and imagine the movement. If you are experiencing pain, the learning becomes associated with pain, and then the lessons are not as useful. It's actually more effective to do a smaller movement that allows you to pay attention than to do a large, painful movement.

For people who find it difficult to read and move at the same time these sequences are also available as free audio downloads from my Web site: www.laviniaplonka.com. When you see an exercise that is followed by the symbol ☽ , just log on, follow the instructions, and you will be able to do the lesson hands-free.

This lesson is best done without shoes. However, if you must wear shoes, make sure they are flexible (like running shoes) and without a hard heel. Take a few minutes to walk around. What do you notice about your walk? What is the sound of your heels striking the ground? The length of your stride? What part of your foot is the last to leave the ground? What do you feel in your back, your arms? What does your pelvis do? If you could step outside yourself and take a look, what kind of person would you see?

In a workshop held on a college campus in the Midwest, Marie spoke about the need to have a particular body language when walking through New York City. I asked volunteers to demonstrate their city walks. I then asked the class to choose who would most likely get mugged. Unanimously the group chose Marie. Her hunched shoulders and crossed arms limited the use of her arms and would have inhibited both running and self-defense. She couldn't turn freely, so her eyes were wide, like prey, looking from side to side. Her pelvis was so tight it would be easy to knock her off balance and grab her purse. She was absolutely shocked. She had no idea that the signal she was sending was the opposite of her intentions.

Stop walking and stand with your feet as parallel as is comfortable. Begin rising up on the balls of your feet, then dropping your heels down to the floor. Try this movement over and over, as if you were bouncing the floor, trying to get the attention of the people on a lower flower. Keep your legs and ankles relaxed. If you feel stress or pain, then lighten up. None of these movement sequences should cause pain. Instead of trying to push yourself, do less and less until it feels absolutely effortless to rise up and drop down on your heels. Then walk around the room again. Pause and rest. You can sit down, lie down, or just stand a moment. You can rest at any time.

Place your weight on your right leg and just bounce your left heel. Leave the bounce and walk. Then do the same thing bouncing your right heel. In between each exploration walk a short time without doing anything special.

Leave the heel and try lifting your toes. Not the whole ball of the foot—just the five toes. Notice if they all come off the floor equally. Can you lift the big toe a little less so that your pinky toe can catch up? Try to create the same rhythm with your toes as you did with your heels. And then take another stroll.

Stand still again. Try lifting the front of the right foot up. Leave your heel on the ground and lift the ball and the toes. What happens in your ankle? In your hip? Are you able to lift the foot without having to bend at the waist? Does it hurt? If so, do less. Try it with your other foot. Repeat it many times, like tapping your foot. Then walk around again.

After another pause, lift up the front of both feet and try walking around on your heels. Can you walk on your heels without making all kinds of compensating movements with your torso? What is happening to your hands? Your jaw? Can you avoid crashing down on your heels? Let it go and take another stroll.

Notice if your walk has changed in any way. And then notice how this makes you feel. Are you enjoying your new walk, or does it feel uncomfortable in some way? What happens when you interrupt your habits? Can you go back easily to your old walk? What does your old walk tell you about yourself? What are some things in this new walk worth exploring?

Take a few minutes after this sequence to jot down your impressions, your reactions, and your observations. During the next few days see if you can remember to notice what your walk feels like—as you cross a room, walk to an appointment, or greet a friend. See if you can discover your relationship to your legs and feet.

TOWARD A NEW YOU

Each of the following chapters includes exercises that invite you to integrate an aspect of body language into your daily interactions. In this way you can begin to shift toward an image that is more congruent with the person you wish to be.

There is an Iroquois saying that you cannot understand a man until you have walked a mile in his moccasins. One of the best ways to start to find a walk of power is to experience how others walk. Here are some possibilities:

- Ask a loved one for permission, then observe them and then try their walk on for size.
- As you walk down a street or through the mall, casually follow someone until you have a sense of his or her walk. Then try it on for a block or two.

- Take note of someone at a party and try their walk on for size while continuing to engage with others.
- Observe someone at work and then try his or her walk when you are alone.
- Exchange walks with a friend.

You will experience two important effects: First, you will literally understand something new about this other person you are observing. Second, by varying your own habitual walk you will discover that your walk changes and improves along with your awareness. You are beginning to develop your sixth sense and are on the road toward your own more potent walk.

Exploration Checklist

- ☐ Experiment with the nine positions of the legs.
- ☐ Observe your walk.
- ☐ Try the movement lesson "The Mechanics of Walking."
- ☐ Write down your impressions of your walk.
- ☐ Practice putting yourself in someone else's shoes in the "Toward a New You" exercise.

Five

GIVING AND RECEIVING—
THE ARMS AND HANDS

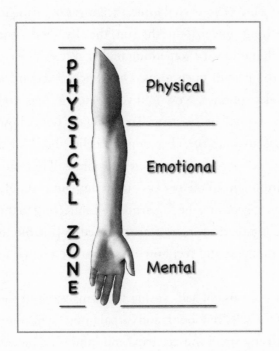

My arms accept and reject what is
offered. What am I receiving? What
am I refusing?

My hands help me think and show
others my thoughts. Where do I find
my hands most often?

EMBRACING, DEFENDING, SUPPORTING

The arms, like the legs, do the work around the house—they clean, hammer, lift, reach.
The upper arms are the physical part of the physical zone, the biceps and triceps pushing

the piano and lifting the baby. The forearms are the emotional part and the direction of the forearms indicates the direction of your emotional attention. Think of reaching to your lover, putting your hands on your hips, or accusing someone angrily—each time your forearm is either going away or coming in toward you.

Is getting up in the morning and lifting your arms up in a glorious stretch merely to wake yourself up? We use our arms so often that we take them for granted—yet they are eloquent in relation to the task at hand. Many gestures are connected to the hands, but for the moment let's just examine how the direction and use of the arms is expressive in itself. Lifting the arms involves the use of your vital force, the power of lifting in the upper arms. The forearms are reaching upward—to the sun, the sky, God—the object of attention is away from yourself and toward something higher. We even have an expression for this—to greet something with open arms. Outstretched toward a puppy or a lover, an extended arm speaks volumes. Now fold your arms. Where you fold your arms—across the chest, the waist—will be discussed later. For now notice how folding your ams brings everything back to yourself. The common belief that folded arms indicate a person is closed or tense is not always completely accurate. There are many factors involved—from the environment to the person's face. But you certainly can know that the person's focus is their interior life, the forearms are connecting to the self. Now put your hands on your hips. Again, the forearms are directed to you, but in a completely different way. Play for a moment and feel how these two are related to aspects of self image.

Many arm injuries are the result of poor use of self—using the arms without the support of or connection with the rest of the self. Tendonitis and carpal tunnel syndrome are both inflammations caused by overusing small muscle areas and inhibiting bigger muscles in the back. Sometimes this is the result of posture, sometimes poor work habits. Both of these can often be connected to emotional tensions—resentment at having to work all day, obsessiveness about getting the job done, insecurity about being a good athlete, and so on.

It is very easy to blame the job or the activity for the injury instead of examining the habits of a lifetime that can be causing the pain. That would mean taking responsibility for the way you are. But I have seen over and over again that once a person becomes interested in herself and begins to study the various holdings that have affected her posture, the improvements can be quite rapid. This can literally create changes in a person's life—suddenly, the dead end job is just that, and you walk away from it, or you find that you are not who you were pretending to be.

Nancy originally came to see me because her left arm and shoulder had been bothering her for months after a seemingly minor injury lifting groceries. She freely admitted that she was now protecting the area and knew that that could be creating more tension in the rest of her body. As we began our work, she also began to tell me about pain she was feeling in her hips, back, and even her legs. Nancy is a short, round woman and she walked like a box with legs. Everything on top was held tightly in, as if she was afraid that if she relaxed her parts would fall off. She gestured wildly with her arms, but her torso never moved, indicating that everything moved from the bicep/tricep area. I could see how the slightest wrong move could result in an arm injury.

After a lesson one day Nancy stood up and walked. Her hips swayed and her shoulders moved. "Woohoo. This could be trouble!" she exclaimed. She sashayed around the room, then sat down heavily and poured out a tale of having been a voluptuous young woman. "But it always got me into trouble." She shook her head. "I just stopped it all—the hips, the shoulders, I rounded over to hide my boobs. I became a blob."

She started wearing makeup and figure-accenting clothing. Her footsteps became lighter as her torso began to conduct the force of her step more elegantly. What did all this have to do with her left shoulder? We could make dozens of connections with Nancy's life and her shoulder: the fact that she used her right hand for everything, which constantly left her left arm in the role of support, the tension in her shoulder girdle, which was compounded by her inflexibility while engaging in physically demanding tasks, and the gripping we discovered in her right buttock and sacrum area that compromised the cross-lateral relationships between right hip and left shoulder. As Nancy slowly unfolded from walking granite to an earth goddess, a lifetime of pain melted away. In the process Nancy's entire attitude—toward men, friends, possibilities changed. All because of a sore arm.

SHOULDER TO THE WHEEL

To be articulate also means to be "jointed." Each joint in the body also articulates aspects of the emotional life. Delsarte called the shoulders the thermometer of the passions. The degree of the articulation of the shoulder indicates the level of emotion—be it joy or grief—that is expressed. This is how we can recognize the difference between a noncommittal shrug and someone overcome with grief, sinking her head between raised shoulders.

The shoulder bears responsibility—the ability to respond—from lifting objects to mobilizing the arms for protection. The term "to shoulder responsibility" can be taken literally. For eons humans literally bore burdens on their backs. Using their shoulders to heave, the shoulder girdle to support, people carried their crops, their water poles, their children, their entire homes. This job has been taken away from most Western shoulders over the last century. Now the weight of financial insecurity, workaholism, family stress, and much more are the burdens that we shoulder. Many people walk around with their shoulders up by their ears. Or one shoulder is higher than the other. For many people the muscles are so tight the top of the shoulder girdle—the area across the top of yourself, comprising your clavicles (collarbones) and scapulae (shoulder blades)—feels like a rock hard surface, almost like bone. What is it that the shoulders are carrying? What would happen if the shoulders let go of carrying the weight of the world?

Sometimes this sense of holding up the world is actually a holding up of yourself. There are a number of reasons for this phenomenon. The Startle Reflex is an instinct we are born with. When you lose your balance, are falling, or hear a loud sound, your entire body reacts and then moves to protect you from danger. If you've ever been working in a quiet room and suddenly you hear a loud door slam, that jump is the startle reflex in action. Part of the startle reflex involves a raising of the shoulders—both as a protective mechanism (protecting the viscera) as well as an auxiliary move to literally hold you up. This movement can become habitual from childhood ("Watch out Johnny, you'll fall!") and sometimes it just gets stuck that way. People locked in this version of the startle reflex communicate a sense of tension and weakness simultaneously. And for good reason—when the shoulders are frozen and up, effective movement of the arms and torso is compromised, creating fertile ground for injury. Raised or rigid shoulders inhibit the ability of the head to turn and compromise effective breathing, leading to even greater tension. Remember Marie's New York City walk.

The placement of the head often affects the shoulders—again, the shoulders bear responsibility. This time they're trying to hold the head up. Whether the head is jutting forward because of years in front of a computer screen, a postural habit formed in childhood, or the result of chronic nearsightedness, this unbalance at the top of the spine makes the shoulders feel a need to rescue the head from collapsing on the chest. This level of tension creates a kind of "turtle" effect. The tension involved in this posture, as well as the limitations it creates for mobility and global vision, make such a person seem timid and defensive at the same time.

Many people say to me, "I try to get my shoulders down, but thirty seconds later I look in the mirror and they've creeped back up again." This is an indication that holding the shoulders has become a postural habit. Often the shoulder girdle has become the "center of gravity" for this person's posture. Instead of moving from the pelvic girdle, which is the center of the body, the shoulder girdle has decided to become the support system. This can happen as the result of the startle reflex, or a back injury, or even sexual trauma, all of which could cut one off from sensation in the pelvis.

Freeing the Shoulder

Even if you think you know how you hold your shoulders, take a moment to sense how they are. Close your eyes and imagine a line going from your right ear to your right shoulder. Now another line from your left ear to your left shoulder. Are they the same length? Does one shoulder feel more forward than another? If you wish to verify, stand for a moment in front of your mirror and notice—is one shoulder higher than the other? Is it the one you imagined? Sometimes your body image is

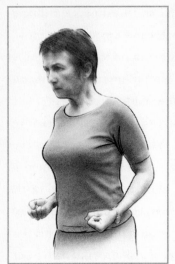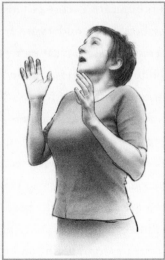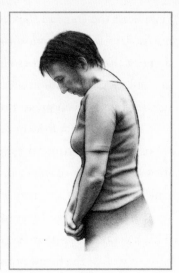

Some examples of shoulders expressing emotions

the exact opposite of what it really is! Even the slightest deviation from being directly centered requires tension. If the shoulders are not just hanging from the skeleton, there is a chronic state of tension somewhere in the shoulder girdle. Even if you are not aware of it on a daily basis, you are communicating something about your insecurities, your stress level, your lack of ease in the way you hold your shoulders. Now take a walk around, and as you walk notice what your arms are doing. Do they swing differently from each other? Are they still? What movement do you feel in your shoulders? What movement do you feel in your pelvis? Don't try to make anything happen—just notice. Before continuing, you may want to write down your impressions for further study.

Sit comfortably in a chair with your feet flat on the floor. Place your hands in your lap with your palms up. Your arms should be loose and slightly bent. Now very slowly begin to raise your right shoulder. This is a slow motion movement—the slower you can do this movement, the more benefit you will receive from it. If you do the movement too quickly, you will just use the same shoulder muscles that you use in your daily life. But if you really slow it down, you can begin to sense the muscles in your back and in your shoulder blade area, for example. Once your shoulder has gone up as high as it can go comfortably, lower it down just as slowly. This is more challenging than it might seem at first attempt, so do it several times. Notice if your shoulder raises and lowers smoothly, or if there are occasional jumps or skips. Don't try to speed past those—just keep going slowly. Does your shoulder go up and down in a straight line, or does it dance around a little? Notice your breathing. Sometimes when we concentrate we unconsciously hold our breath. See if you can keep breathing as you do these movements and notice whether you always inhale and exhale with the same movement. In other words, do you always inhale when your shoulder goes up, or down? If you notice a pattern, feel free to experiment. What does it feel like to try the opposite breath? Or even to breathe in a random pattern, completely different from the movement? Now the next time you raise your right shoulder up, hold it there for a moment. Keep breathing. But keep your shoulder up near your ear somewhere. Is this easy? Familiar? This is where many people live, with one or both shoulders in a constant state of tension. Now once again slowly lower your shoulder. Sit back and relax a moment. And notice. Does your shoulder feel different in any way? Let your thoughts wander for a minute—where do they go?

Try the same movement with your left shoulder. With your eyes closed, see if you can picture the movements that you did on the right side. What you are doing is clarifying what you have just experienced. Keep your breath soft as you picture raising and lowering your left shoulder. After a few minutes of imagining, begin to actually raise your left shoulder toward your ear. And lower it down. As you repeat this movement, notice if it feels different than you imagined it or different from the right side. You already may have forgotten what the right side feels like. And the right side might feel different now than when you began. So just notice what stands out for you as you do this movement. It's the noticing that's important—not trying to make things even.

When you finish, take a rest. Then get up and walk around, noticing if there is anything new about your walk or your stance.

What Are You Shouldering?

Make a list of all the things you are shouldering. Can you find some new ways to approach these responsibilities? What does it mean to be "response-able"? Do you have to hunch yourself and shoulder your way through life? Do you have to bear the entire burden? Are there some burdens you can let go of? Or perhaps carry differently? Give yourself a few times during the day to notice your shoulders. You can set specific times (some people set an alarm on their watches or computers) to remind you to notice. Or you can use certain situations or people as reminders (the obnoxious office mate, your child, the phone ringing). This can be both very challenging and very rewarding. Play around with other shoulder metaphors. I have always been fascinated with the attitudes of the shoulders and the word *should*. Even though they are not linguistically connected, I have often observed people using that word as their shoulders rise. Give yourself time each night to write down your impressions—without judgment.

HANDS DOWN, THUMBS UP

Gesture is parallel to the impression received;
it is, therefore, always anterior to speech.

François Delsarte

Delsarte believed that our hands are indicative of our mental process. Contemporary science bears out his intuition again. Stuart Wilcox, an evolutionary linguist and specialist in sign language, has speculated that "language emerged through bodily action before becoming codified in speech." The neural connection between the hands and the brain has been firmly established. In fact, science says that our hands *are* our thoughts revealed. Linguist David McNeill calls gesture a *"form* of thought—not just an expression of thought, but 'cognitive being' itself." Studies have shown that when we gesture with the hands, we are not gesturing in order to help the listener, but we actually are assisting and clarifying our own mental process. The gesture is an essential part of formation of thoughts. When used intentionally, the hands emphasize your point. When used unconsciously, they often betray your thoughts. Every action of the hand—from pressing palms together to the position of your thumb while shaking hands tells a story. Suddenly shoving your hands in your pockets at an awkward moment makes sense. You're hiding your thoughts!

Bring your palms toward each other slowly, but stop just before touching. Move them closer and farther away several times. As you do this, you may experience a sense of stickiness that seems to want to connect them. The Chinese call this *chi* and use it in their martial and healing arts. From a Western perspective, we can look at the electrochemical process that takes place at nerve endings. The human organism is a great conductor of electricity—the evil robots in the movie *The Matrix* used humans for battery power! When you bring your hands together you are creating a closed circuit and also sending a huge amount of neurological information to the sensory part of your brain. You could say you are bringing your thoughts together. When you see someone tapping their fingertips together, you know they are forming a thought. Many religions and cultures use the gesture of bringing the palms together. Something about connecting/collecting the self and directing the fingers upward sends our thoughts to something greater. Compare that with bringing the palms together and interlacing your fingers—suddenly the gesture becomes all about you—you're bringing the fingers back to yourself.

Delsarte classified the various functions of the hand:

1. To define or indicate—e.g., pointing
2. To affirm or deny—hand moving up and down or sideways
3. To mold or detect—fingers softly coming apart and together
4. To conceal or reveal—closing and opening fist
5. To surrender or hold—open palm or cupped palm

6. To accept or reject—palm beckons or palm pushes away

7. To inquire or acquire—hand reaches or pulls inward

8. To support or protect—palm up or covering

9. To caress or attack—to stroke or slap

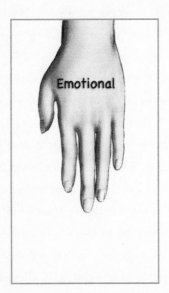
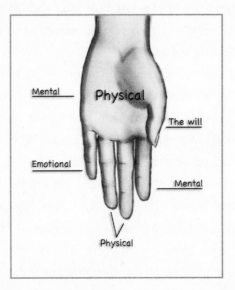

By looking at the zones illustrated above that the hand is divided into, you can begin to experiment with these nine classes of gesture.

The front, or palm, is the vital zone. This is where the majority of nerve endings for your sense of touch are located. When you reach out in the dark, you touch the light switch with the palm side of your hand. The palm is also the area that connects with the pot handle, the hammer, the rungs of the ladder. It is the working part of the hand. When you put your hand out in the "stop" gesture, you are presenting your vital energy against an approaching force. Shaking hands originated as a signal of "I come in peace." If your hand is holding someone else's hand, neither one of you is going to reach for a weapon (unless you're left handed!).

Some scholars have postulated that we developed right and left handedness so that the right hand could hold the sword to attack while the left hand held the shield to protect. According to the ancients, the two sides of the body symbolize our own duality. The right side was light, male, intellect, action. The left side was dark, female, intuitive, receptive. Much like the Chinese yin and yang, the body was seen as a reflection of all the forces in the cosmos. Along the way, however, certain groups decided that qualities like femininity and darkness were linked to evil. The left hand became associated with the "dark side." Left handers in Western culture were punished and "reeducated." To this day, lower-caste Indians sweep floors with their left hand behind their back, and several cultures never eat with the left hand. The English word sinister *traces its roots back to the Latin, where it means both on the left as well as unlucky.*

There are theories that connect the functions of the hand to the opposing brain hemisphere—i.e., the left-handed person is right-brain dominant, and vice versa. But one must be careful not to generalize because there are many other factors at play in observing one's use of the hands. One of the most important is to remember that we live in a right-handed world. Door knobs and appliances are all designed for the right-handed person, so a lefty naturally adapts. In terms of observing body language, it is interesting to notice the kinds of gestures your different hands makes. You may observe that, literally, one hand doesn't know what the other hand is doing.

The back of the hand is the emotional part. Remember the archaic custom of kissing a lady's hand? Imagine the reaction if the gentleman turned the lady's palm upward and kissed her palm. That would be a powerful sexual statement that certainly would have raised eyebrows and temperatures in Victorian society. Try stroking your cheek with the palm of your hand. Then turn your hand over and do the same with the back of your hand. Is there a difference in the way you tilt your head? In even the quality of how you stroke? Even of which cheek you prefer to touch? This is not to say that you only feel emotions when using the back of the hand. As I mentioned earlier, at each moment four things are happening—sensing, thought, emotions, and movement. The hand shows us what predominates in the mind.

The side of the hand is the mental part. People use the side of the hand to define a point—think of a chopping motion or a sideways sweep of the hand that says, "That's enough!" Think of the difference between a military salute and the placement of your hand in the Pledge of Allegiance.

Even the fingers have different zones and functions. You wouldn't point or indicate with your middle finger, for example. You could say, "Well of course, that feels weird." But why? The nerve endings of the different fingers fire different parts of the brain. Touching something that you are familiar with fires completely different areas of the brain than touching something new. And if someone touches *you,* it fires another completely different area. Based on his observations, Delsarte divided the fingers in the following fashion:

The index finger is mental. You use it to make a point, to indicate.

The middle and ring finger together are physical. Your middle finger, being the longest, reaches out to touch things first. In classical theater the middle finger was actually called "the sense of touch." You can often see paintings of nymphs or dancers delicately extending the middle finger toward a flower.

The pinky is emotional. From Dr. Evil in *Austin Powers* to that wonderful expression, "I've got him wrapped around my little finger," we can sense the emotion in the pinky.

The thumb is a class of its own. According to Delsarte, it expresses a person's will, energy, and interests. In death the thumb is tucked in. In ancient Rome thumbs up meant the gladiator lives; thumbs down, he's dead. We've all experienced varying levels of handshakes and have wondered why a limp handshake gives us the creeps. Without the commitment of the thumb, the grip has no vitality.

Indian mudras are a complex series of hand gestures with symbolic significance. In many ways, their meanings correspond to our contemporary gestures and to studies of the hand's neural connections to the sensory cortex. They also have some interesting parallels to Delsarte's theories. For example, the thumb symbolizes all things divine and the index finger your individual self. Your thumb therefore indicates your relationship to spirit or higher energy. The index finger is "you." When you point to someone and say, "You, come here," you don't point with the pinky. The Vitarka mudra—bringing your thumb to your index finger—is called the "cognition of instruction gesture." It means "I got it."—exactly like the way you would gesture "A—OK!"

Listening to the Hand ❥

Try the following exercise using your dominant hand first. Then give yourself a couple of days before trying the second hand.

Lie comfortably on your back—you can have your legs long, your knees bent, or even prop your legs up on a bolster. If it is not possible to lie on your back, sit with your dominant elbow on a desk or some cushions in your lap. If you are lying down, make sure that your head is comfortable—not too high or too low. Bring your dominant arm horizontally out to the side on the floor so that it is at a 90-degree angle from your torso. Now bend the arm so that your forearm is in the air at a 90-degree angle from your upper arm. Where is your hand in relation to the forearm? Are the fingers pointing to the ceiling, or is the wrist relaxed with the fingers drooping toward the floor? Very, very slowly, begin moving your hand. If your fingers are reaching skyward, slowly let them melt, let the wrist droop. If your fingers are drooping, slowly, slowly let them curl upward, bringing your palm to face the front. Repeat this movement several times. Go extremely slowly so that you can feel where your hand moves smoothly and where the hand wants to jump and skip to another part of the movement. Notice what it feels like as you slowly uncurl and curl your fingers. Do the fingers separate? Are they touching each other?

As I mentioned before, many hand and arm injuries are related to tensions and constraints in the shoulder and back area. You can begin to sense your gripping when you do this exercise slowly with attention.

Notice your breathing, what you feel in your neck and your shoulder blades. Do this movement about ten times, and then rest by putting your arm down by your side.

Bring your arm back to the same position. Let your wrist droop down. Begin to move your index finger around by itself. Just feel what it's like to separately move the finger. Then continue with each finger in turn—notice which fingers separate easily, where they move, the quality of the movement. Now slowly begin to turn your hand so that your fingers point once to you and once away, as if your hand was gently being blown by a breeze. Notice how far your hand can turn easily in each direction. Rest.

Resume the same position and let your wrist droop down. Slowly bring the tip of your pinky to touch the tip of your thumb and repeat several times. How does it feel to touch your thumb? Now try the other way. Bring the tip of your thumb over to touch your pinky. How is that different from the pinky touching the thumb? Or is it exactly the same? What do the other three fingers do—are they bent or straight? Slowly, keeping the thumb and pinky connected, try bending and straightening the three fingers. Now bring the hands to vertical and try the same thing, bending and straightening the other three fingers. Rest.

Notice what this arm feels like in comparison to the other arm. Sense each hand. Roll to your side and come to standing and see if anything attracts your attention as being different.

Learning to study the tensions in your hands and listening to how they echo in your shoulders and back can be a revelation. It can change how you reach, write, shrug, and more. You actually may find that the word is truly at your fingertips.

TALKING WITH YOUR HANDS

Suddenly an entire vista of meaning has opened. The hands become a code to the thoughts and feelings of the people we are interacting with. Begin to notice what you do and what others do with their hands. And see if you can at the same moment catch what you're thinking or feeling or what others are trying to express. Are the palms together, fingers curled, fingertips tapping, back of the hand to the cheek? Begin to write down the gestures and positions you remember as well as your gut response to them—both your own and others'. See if you can observe your own unconscious gestures, as this is a doorway to beginning to understand how your unconscious thoughts form your perceptions of the world and other people's perceptions of you.

Create a list of gestures—use separate pages for you and those you observe. You may discover that you suddenly notice in yourself a gesture you had observed in someone else. As you increase your awareness you'll notice you have habitual gestures and occasional ones. When you catch yourself repeating a gesture, make a mark next to it—you can even add a note about it. Or if you catch yourself making someone else's gesture, note that as well. You will notice that some gestures include other parts of the body, such as the face and the chest. You can make a note of these gestures and record your impressions. As we go more deeply into the study of these parts, the meanings of these kinds of gestures will become more clear.

TOWARD A NEW YOU

Do your hands and arms betray or support you? What signals are you sending to others? Here are some experiments.

- Based on some of the above exercises, choose two gestures you use a lot, such as folding your arms, rubbing your mouth, or tapping your fingers. Each time you catch yourself in this gesture/posture, intentionally change it. Change it to anything. If your hands are in your pockets, take them out. If they are cupping your chin, put them down. Notice what happens with the person you are speaking with.
- Using the same two gestures or two others, try to exaggerate what you already are doing following the yes. If you're scratching your nose, scratch faster. If

your shoulders are up, lift them higher. Be careful not to do this while talking to your boss! Notice what is happening inside. Do this for only about fifteen seconds, then drop the exercise entirely.

- Intentionally change your handshake.
- If you feel nervous—first date, meeting with a new client—take a moment to bring your thoughts together. Bring your hands together gently in the prayer position, or just spend a moment allowing your fingertips to touch each other. If you're in a public place, you can even just let the fingertips of one hand softly touch the thumb tip a few times. Connect it to an easy breath. Then step in the door.

Exploration Checklist

☐ Try the movement lesson "Freeing the Shoulder."

☐ What are you shouldering? Make a list of your response-abilities.

☐ Using Delsarte's nine categories, try intentionally creating various hand gestures. Find sentences or phrases that go with those gestures.

☐ Do the movement sequence "Listening to the Hand."

☐ Talking with your hands—make a list of your gestures and other people's gestures. Mark the ones you repeat or that bother you.

☐ Experiment with ways to empower your gestures in the "Toward a New You" exercises.

Six

THE HEART OF THE MATTER—
THE CHEST

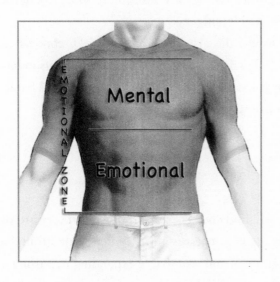

My chest is a trunk filled with emotions
    as well as organs. What is locked in
    my trunk? What needs to open?
My solar plexus is like the sun in myself.
    Is it shining, or is it crushed?
My breath is my life. Am I starving
    myself? Why?

THE TRUTH CENTER

In theater there is a saying, "The chest does not lie," which implies that your true
emotional state is reflected in the carriage of your chest. Unconsciously we are both

communicating and reading other people's emotions in sometimes subtle but sometimes large shifts in the chest. The rib cage surrounds several vital organs and the movement of the rib cage affects the quality of breath, flexibility in the back, even the timber and strength of a voice. For the last two hundred years science and medicine has insisted that the organs in the torso are merely mechanical devices, pumps and bellows that keep the human machine running. The idea that our emotional life is somehow connected to these physiological functions has been ridiculed. And yet we might describe someone as walking around with his chest puffed up, or you might have a gut feeling. Neurotransmitters have been found in the stomach, indicating that a gut feeling may be a kind of intelligence that informs the thinking brain. And as mentioned earlier, new discoveries in the field of neurocardiology are prompting some to call the heart another brain, the seat of the emotional intelligence.

From Homer to Shakespeare to Disney, the arts celebrate the deep connection between the emotions and the chest. While science may have forgotten or misunderstood its importance, our kinesthetic sense has always been there for us to see, as Saint-Exupéry's Little Prince once said, "Not just with the eyes, but with the heart."

How Do You Feel?

Find your neutral stance. Where do you find your chest right now? Is it forward or in back of the plumb line? Is this where your chest is all the time? Walk around a little bit and experiment with the position of your chest. Try expanding it, puffing it out. How does that affect the rest of your walk? How do you feel? Sink your chest in and down, as if you had pushed all the air out of your lungs. Walk around a bit like this and notice what comes up.

Many people are afraid to experience different postures, especially in the chest, so it is particularly important to give yourself a little time to let this posture sink in.

As you go through your day, see if you can catch moments when you are interacting with someone—maybe lunch with a friend or a business conversation. See if your chest is saying anything. Take the time to write down your observations and see—does your chest have a particular repertoire, or is it frozen on one plane?

Kevin was a particularly pompous and arrogant man who took my course in order to debunk me. Every time we did an exercise like this, he went out of his way to make sure everyone saw how stupid they appeared. When we would try the positions of the torso, he would just sit and smirk at the rest of the class. Kevin considers himself an educated intellectual who is only interested in the facts. One day during a partner exercise, his part-ner told him that walking with her chest depressed made her feel depressed. She asked Kevin to try it. He did a mocking exaggeration of her posture and said loudly, "I feel like a jerk." The rest of the class stopped and stood quietly looking at him. He never returned. I always felt bad for Kevin because his own rigidity imprisoned not only his ability to learn, but his possibility to have a greater repertoire for expression and relationship. But he had, indeed, expressed his own truth—he felt like a jerk, and everyone had silently agreed.

INSPIRATION, ASPIRATION, RESPIRATION

When you inhale, you literally are feeding yourself. The human organism can go weeks without food. In fact, there are people in India who claim they haven't eaten in a year. They call themselves breatharians and insist that they derive nutrition directly from the sun. We can go days without water but only a few minutes without air. Of course you must be breathing, or you wouldn't be reading this—yet, *how* you breathe affects your physical and emotional states, just as those states can affect how you breath.

Delsarte placed the lungs in the mental zone of the emotional center. His rationale was connected to the Hindu idea that breath is connected to energy or spirit. To be in-spired is suddenly to be filled with some magnificent idea—the original Latin means "to blow air into," or "to breathe in." And to aspire literally means to "breathe desire to-ward." The breath and emotion are inextricably linked. Susana Bloch's Alba Emoting Method stresses that a key aspect of emotional expression is the respiratory pattern. Something of exquisite beauty can literally take your breath away. A woman with a breathless or breathy voice gives the impression of weakness and fragility. We take a big breath when we're about to do something physically demanding.

Yet one of the biggest hidden culprits in contemporary culture is the constant need to hold the breath. Everyone is waiting for the other shoe to drop. Holding the breath is a primitive instinct—a self-protective mechanism to hide from a predator. But we have become so anxiety driven that we hold our breath while passing another car, while pouring hot water, while waiting for our child to get off the bus, when the phone rings. All this breath holding affects our physiology and psychology. The rib cage becomes immobile. I have worked with students who react in shock when they learn that the ribs *can* move. Many people have been told that abdominal breathing is the proper way to breathe, completely ignoring all the other parts of the skeleton that participate in the act of breathing. Imagine a lion or an opera singer breathing with just the abdomen—it would completely diminish their power. Since your ribs are connected to the spine, immobile ribs contribute to tension in the spine. And once the ribs are "stuck," breath-ing becomes even more difficult.

Inhibited breath creates a number of different situations that affect your body lan-guage, and your body language can also affect your breath.

Dennis told me about a faculty meeting at his school where someone had proposed start-ing a program he was uncomfortable with. "I sat there and folded my arms across my chest as I listened to the proposal. I don't think it's a habitual posture for me, but as the other teacher talked, I felt myself full of resistance to his idea. All of a sudden I realized that my arms were holding my chest so tightly that I was barely breathing. I put my arms down by my sides and instantly felt more air coming in. As my ability to breathe increased, I was literally better able to take in his idea, let it move around in me."

The lack of full oxygenation can exacerbate pain in diseases like fibromyalgia. Poor breathing patterns can affect sleep, making an individual sensitive and cranky. This toxicity can make the body and the individual seem rigid and fragile at the same time. It is difficult to be spontaneous or to move freely if the chest is held. This tension affects the relation of the arms to the big muscles in the back, so there isn't a lot of power in lifting or pushing, making the person seem even weaker and more prone to arm injuries. Many times the chest begins to sink in, with the front muscles of the upper chest actually contracting and pulling the person downward. Then the struggle for verticality goes to the back and head. In what becomes a vicious cycle, this posture creates rapid, shallow breaths, which the nervous system then interprets as "you are in danger." Dr. Susana Bloch's research indicates that the respiratory pattern is intimately linked with emotional states. The nervous system uses the breath as information. Deep, easy breaths trigger different chemicals than rapid, ragged breaths or inhibited breath. In *The Potent Self,* Feldenkrais says, "Many people hold their breath in one way or another. The body image they have formed is such that they have to produce a preparatory rearrangement of their throat, chest, and abdomen before they can speak or initiate any motion whatsoever. . . . The normal ventilation is upset, with profound effects on the acid-base balance of the blood." Going back to our animal roots, an animal who doesn't breathe fully doesn't have a lot of options for flight or fight. It will be overtaken and destroyed.

Your breathing pattern affects others as well—the natural tendency of organisms to entrain, to adopt the rhythms of those around them, is easily influenced by the breath. A shallow breather can make an entire room anxious. It also betrays lack of confidence so that no matter what you are saying, you will be hard to listen to.

> She with one breath attunes the spheres,
> And also my poor human heart.
> HENRY DAVID THOREAU

The Breath of Life ⟩

There are many wonderful books and tapes that explore breathing, the virtues of proper oxygenation, and the various ways to improve it. This exercise is designed to help you identify the parts of yourself that move or don't move when you breathe in a relaxed state. It is not a lesson to teach you the proper way to breathe, since every situation in life requires a different kind of breathing pattern. This exercise is intended to provide some insights into muscular holdings that communicate qualities and emotions to both yourself and others.

Find a comfortable position—it can be lying down, on your back or your side, or sitting up in a chair. Just listen to your breath for a few minutes. Don't try to change anything. Just notice. What moves as you breathe? Our breathing patterns are different at rest than in activity, so just listen to how you are at rest. Notice the length of your inhale. Notice the length of your exhale. Notice the pauses in between the inhale and the exhale. Is one longer than the other? They may be different; they may be the same. Just notice your pattern.

Place your hand on your abdomen and notice if there is any movement there. Then see if you can continue breathing for a few minutes keeping your abdomen still. Don't let it move. If you are primarily an abdominal breather, this can be challenging, so listen to your comfort and safety level. As you breathe in this fashion, what do you feel? Just notice—emotions come up quickly when you work with your breath. Now remove your hand and breathe normally. Notice what your breathing feels like now.

Now place your hand on your chest. A good place is in the area of the sternum (breastbone). Notice any movement you feel there. The chest moves more when we are engaged in an aerobic activity (picture how profoundly the chest moves in a sprinter at the end of the race), but there is still some rise and fall at rest. Now intentionally inhibit the movement of your chest. Even if it felt like you were not moving there in the first place, purposely hold your chest and ribs in place. Let everything else that wants to move do so. Is this a familiar or uncomfortable experience? Notice again: What predominates? Thoughts? Sensations? Emotions? Resume your habitual breathing and notice what that is like.

Explore other parts of your torso—you can inhibit movement in the back, shoulders, and clavicles.

BREATH AND SPIRIT

Mindfulness of breath is a principle tenet of many meditative practices. The Buddhist tradition stresses the receiving and letting go process that takes place with every breath. "I breathe in relinquishment, I breathe out relinquishment . . ." Hindus use many exercises with the breath in their yogic practice: one of the branches of yoga is called Pranayama. (The word *prana* in Sanskrit means both *breath* and *spirit*.) The practice is designed to bring both physical and spiritual vitality to the student. In Chinese philosophy *chi* is a term that connotes both spirit, the vital energy of the body, and the breath. Christian tradition speaks of the breath of the Holy Spirit. In all of these approaches we can see the link between the action of the breath and the action of the mind. While the aim of these meditative practices is not so much improved function as a deeper quality of attention, one of the side benefits meditation students experience is better health—reduced stress, better cardiac function, and more vitality.

What Are You Waiting For?

At various moments in the day—whether they be stressful or ordinary—pause and notice the breath. What emotions are behind the pattern? Are you waiting to exhale or inhale? What is your posture? If possible, record your impressions on the following chart when you catch yourself. Then set aside a time during the week to catalog your findings. You can also download a copy of the chart from www.laviniaplonka.com.

WHAT AM I WAITING FOR?

SITUATION	BREATH QUALITY	EMOTION
_____	_____	_____

Comment:

SITUATION	BREATH QUALITY	EMOTION
_____	_____	_____

Comment:

SITUATION	BREATH QUALITY	EMOTION
_____	_____	_____

Comment:

Here are some examples:

SITUATION	BREATH QUALITY	EMOTION
Picked up phone	Held	Nervous

Comment: I thought it was Jeff and I didn't want to talk to him.

SITUATION	BREATH QUALITY	EMOTION
Writing checks	Shallow	None

Comment: I didn't feel an emotion, but each time I try to balance my checkbook I get the math all wrong.

SITUATION	BREATH QUALITY	EMOTION
Hung up phone	Sigh	Pleasure

Comment: I think I'm in love!

As you become more aware of your breathing patterns, you will become more sensitive to others around you. You will begin to observe when others are anxious, and simply through your own awareness of your breath you will be able to create an atmosphere of comfort around you.

MATTERS OF THE HEART

"Her heart sank." The National Institute for Mental Health posits a direct link between depression and heart problems. Studies have shown that depression increases the risk of heart disease. Can the way you carry your chest eventually affect your health? The metaphors in our culture abound—"He died of a broken heart," or "I'm absolutely heartsick." When a widow of a marine killed in Iraq was interviewed on the radio, she began speaking calmly enough, then said, "It . . . feels like someone has ripped out a piece of my heart." Then she broke down. You can imagine her clutching her chest as she spoke. In the old Latin Mass there was a moment of group contrition. The congregation would intone, "Mea culpa, mea culpa, mea maxima culpa." (My fault, my fault, my huge fault.) As they did, they would hit the left side of their chests with their right fists.

In the other direction, we have expressions like "Her heart leapt at the sight of him coming around the corner." "His heart was in his throat." "His heart fairly leapt out of his chest." Everyone has felt an increased heart rate in a moment of danger or excitement—whether it's the love of your life or an oncoming car. The combination of adrenaline and endorphins in a moment of excitement gets the heart pumping more oxygen-rich blood into a system hepped up by mind-altering neurotransmitters. The result ranges from a rush to heart pounding and trembling. The sympathetic nervous system is charged and ready for action.

In both of the above cases you witness the physiological miracle of the human organism. The heart, brain, and nervous system respond to cues so quickly that your ordinary thoughts can't possibly follow them. You can tell whether someone is happy to see you or in a funk by observing their chest. You can also learn to differentiate a person's mood from his habitual state—for example a politician who generally walks erect with his chest forward will have a different slump if he loses an election, than someone who lives in perpetual self-pity. A mood is transient and shifts across a person's body landscape like a passing cloud. A state is where you find yourself day after day. It is important to pay attention to everything surrounding what you perceive to be a person's state.

Jocelyn walked into my office, the picture of southern charm and elegance. She had pulled up in a late-model Cadillac and was Gucci from her purse to her shoes. She strode in, chest forward, a huge smile on her still pretty face. She was coming to see me because she thought my work could help her daughter. "I'm not here for myself," she said. As we chatted I felt like I was at a debutante ball. Jocelyn's posture was so beyond perfect that I half expected her to break into some kind of song by Doris Day or some other fifties icon.

Somehow it emerged that Jocelyn had back pain. I invited her to walk to see what we could uncover. She stood up, thrust out her chest, pinned back her shoulders, and sashayed across the floor as if she was accepting the crown for Miss America. Her dazzling smile almost belied the incredible tension in her back and jaw. I asked her if she needed to press her chest forward so much. She deflated to a normal posture. "You mean . . . walk like that? But that's bad posture!" As we explored the postural choices available to her, she revealed her deep insecurities—her lack of any skills or talent, her reliance on her good looks, her dreams of being a a film star, which led to a series of humiliating auditions and bit parts that went nowhere, the disastrous marriage, and her new, wealthy but uninteresting husband. "He's fine. He takes care of me. I won't ever starve." We played with what it might be like to face the world without having to press her chest forward. Her back pain disappeared.

SOMETIMES A CIGAR IS . . . JUST A CIGAR

By studying a person's chest you can often determine that person's livelihood. Desk jockeys and computer cowboys are often round-shouldered with a slight slump in the chest, giving a rounded hump in the back (kyphosis). Certain construction workers have their chests expanded in all directions. Dancers often have their chests forward.

You see someone rail thin walking with her chest up, her feet pointing outward, and you think "dancer." You see a powerful man in jeans and a plaid shirt, his face tan from years of exposure, and you don't think, "Ah, a computer programmer." However, their carriage and personae are still the result of choice. There are plenty of construction workers who slump, many office workers with erect backs. When you look at a dancer like Mikhail Baryshnikov, you don't see the cliché body of a dancer. He slouches like a regular guy, smoking his cigarette, then soars through the air as if defying gravity. Is your occupation the result of your self image, and is that self image the result of your attitude and habits?

Some professions require specific body language habits. For example, soccer referees rely on body language—gestures as well as postures and attitudes. Don, a professional soccer referee, told me that an effective referee must have a compassionate yet firm demeanor. When a timid person attempts to referee, his habitual body language interferes with his effectiveness, diluting the power of the hand signals. When a referee's posture has an aggressive quality, he can negatively affect the players and the fans.

Differentiating between a carriage that has been "assumed," a carriage that is the result of repetitive use, and a carriage that is a genuine example of the emotion portrayed is a skill that takes time. When you look at Michael Jordan, you can feel that his actions are congruent with the way he carries himself. As he walks, you know his run is fast, his aim is sure. He is not trying to be an athlete, he *is* an athlete.

Is there tension in the stance? Does the person seem comfortable? Is there an artificiality to the carriage? Does the choice seem to create limitations? For example, going back to the construction worker—is he like a refrigerator with arms, all bulk and no ability to turn, bend, or access his torso? Or does he move with ease and power? Or perhaps somewhere in between? If you look like a dancer, people will relate to you in a certain way. Therefore, assuming this position of the chest in some way reflects a personal choice, although it is often unconscious. Each person is actually a complex pattern of movement.

Olga is a tall, elderly Russian lady living in the deep South. Her hair is always tied in a French twist and her statuesque bearing appears somewhat regal. Yet when she talks she is effusive, giggly, and playful. Her movements are gawky—as if she was an eleven-year-old girl who woke up to find herself a six-foot-tall adult.

One day in class we were talking about the carriage of the chest. A small, timid woman pointed out Olga's carriage as the epitome of elegance, "You sit like a princess. Were you a ballerina?" she asked. Olga was taken aback. "Oh my! I just don't know how to walk any other way! When I was growing up in Russia, my father had very strict rules about how a lady should appear. I always had to walk with my back very, very straight, or I was punished." She reached up and pulled the comb holding her hair up and let it fall down. "And I never, never was allowed to wear my hair down. Only loose women wore their hair down." She tossed her head and giggled. "Now I am sixty years old. Even today when I let my hair down like this I feel like . . . a very bad girl." She immediately put her hair back up.

Olga could have rebelled and become a wild and crazy temptress. Or she could have wilted under her father's sternness, becoming round-shouldered and timid. Olga remained Daddy's girl, eleven years old forever, still pleasing him with her good behavior at age sixty. By just looking at the carriage of her chest, one might come to the conclusion that she was someone regal and elegant when in fact she was just trying to please her father.

SOLAR ENERGY

"It was like a blow to my solar plexus." A real blow to the solar plexus literally can knock you out. This huge ganglion of nerves regulates much nervous system function. Some Hindu texts place the third chakra, the seat of the will, in the solar plexus. And Delsarte placed the emotional part of the emotional center right in this middle area.

Let's return for a moment to our language and its metaphors. "Go ahead, vent your spleen!" "I can't believe she had the gall to say that." "He really galls me." "I just can't stomach it." The British have a saying for someone who is cranky: He is "feeling liverish." And again, "I have a gut feeling."

It's difficult to see a differentiation between the upper chest and lower chest in ordinary observation. However, it is possible to notice if, as a person walks, the area between the sternum (breastbone) and the pelvis moves at all. Often there will be a deep hidden tension, freezing the torso. It's almost as if these people are "holding it all in" or "keeping it together." It's often easier to see this in the spine than in the front. Ulcers and indigestion compete with outbursts of anger. These are often high-performance people whose passion and energy is imprisoned in the fascia and ribs surrounding their vital organs.

The Touch of Emotion

As our hands are extensions of our thoughts, where and how we use them in relation to the chest speak volumes. With a friend or in a mirror, play with placing your hand on the different parts of your chest, and notice what you feel. Alternate with using your open palm and closing your hand into a soft or hard fist so that the backs of the fingers have contact with the chest. Remember that the palm is reflective of your physical self; the back of the hand reflects the emotional. Either cross your arms or place one arm across the chest and the other hand somewhere else. See if thoughts like "Oh my gosh!," "I don't believe it!," "Honest! I mean it!," or "Oh, no!" come up. See if touching different parts of the chest affects the quality of the emotion. Are any of these gestures familiar to you? For example, do you often stand with your arms crossed? Do you tend to drum your fingers on your sternum while thinking? Note down any gestures that either seemed habitual or caused a reaction in you. Take some time to look at pictures of both yourself and others and note where the hands and arms are in relation to the chest.

THE HIDDEN DIMENSION

In our frontally oriented culture we forget the eloquence of the back—until it hurts. Yet how the back shapes the front is key in our observations of ourselves and others. Often you can recognize a friend from behind, which means that person has a distinctive language in her carriage. The ribs hang from the spine, so the relationship of the spine to a person's emotional expression is inextricable. Entire books have been written about the many properties of the spine—addressing posture, metaphor, injuries, strengthening, even what yogis call *kundalini* energy, a flame of energy that travels upward from the tailbone. All physical disciplines—from yoga to the martial arts to sports—emphasize the primacy of awareness of the spine. If you suffer from back pain, you can be sure that it affects how your entire skeleton moves and therefore how others perceive you. Learning to view yourself in three dimensions can allow you to see the hidden tensions that are connected to unexpressed rage, fear, and sorrow.

If you look at paintings throughout history, from Jesus Christ and the saints to women languidly resting, you will see that many sympathetic subjects sit with the spine curved slightly to one side. Unless they all had scoliosis, there may be a reason for this choice. A straight spine conveys directness, strength, and efficiency, all important qualities. (In fact, we say someone who is weak has no backbone.) But sometimes we need to receive, to be pliable, to surround someone with our draping attention. While bending the spine habitually can result in postural discomfort, listening to your spine and head while engaged in a situation that calls for compassion can be a useful tool, especially when what you are feeling is irritation. In fact, learning to listen to where your back tenses can inform both you and the person you are conversing with.

If you have back pain, explore some of the therapies available to help restore the spine to flexibility. The following exercise is one of many offered by the Feldenkrais Method that explores the relationship of front and back.

The Real You ꒷

This chapter began with the statement "The chest does not lie." Yet many people use their chests to lie. Learning to see the tensions associated with the positions helps us to interpret them. Like Jocelyn covering her insecurities with her Miss America posture, some people's chests tell contradictory stories. An actor may cover his shyness by expanding his chest. Manipulative people may hide their aggression behind a sunken chest, which makes them appear meek. In the theater, we call this working "contra-mask." A smiling, friendly character who suddenly shocks the audience with an evil act is using a contra-mask technique. Our mythology is full of stories about another self hiding behind a disguise. Superman hid his true self behind the façade of Clark Kent. Most people think that the position of the chest is hereditary, or stuck, but like other parts of the self, we have choices. If your chest has become fixed, your ability to respond to different situation is limited and people will make unconscious judgments about your personality and abilities based on their perceptions. The following exercise explores some basic properties of movement of the chest: arching and rounding. Side bending, twisting, and expanding are all qualities that can be explored further in order to better understand your chest both front and back. For this lesson you will need a space on the floor where you feel comfortable lying down, either a carpeted surface or on a mat. If you need a support for your head, have that ready in advance. If getting to the floor and back up is difficult, you can do this sequence lying in bed.

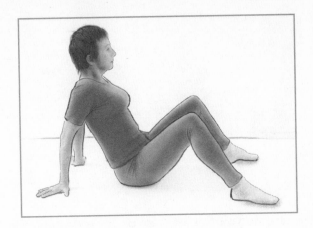

Sit on the floor and lean back on your hands. Bend your knees and bring your feet to standing position.

Now slowly let your knees tilt down to the right, come back up, and then tilt to the left. Do this movement several times and notice if you feel any movement in your chest. Are there moments when your chest changes its position—either reaching forward or rounding back? Or is your chest stable, staying the same the whole time? Which way does your chest prefer to be—rounded, extended, or somewhere in between? How easy is it for you to move your legs?

(Note: If it is impossible for you to sit in this fashion, you can modify this exercise by sitting in a chair and placing your hands on the chair seat behind you. Let your knees and legs travel right and left, keeping your feet in place. The experience in your chest will be more subtle, but you will still feel how your torso responds to your legs.)

Now lie down on your back. Bend your knees and bring your feet to standing position a good distance apart from each other.

Slowly begin tilting your right knee to the left. If you're finding that your leg knocks into the left leg, just move your left leg farther away.

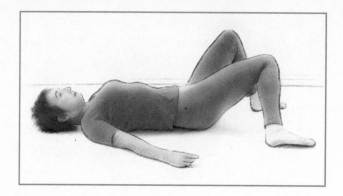

As your leg tilts, do you feel any movement anywhere else? Does your pelvis move? Your torso? Do you feel anything in your chest? What about your breathing? Rest.

Spread your legs. Now put your arms on the floor above your head so that if someone were looking down at you you'd look like a big X.

If your arms won't go that high, just bring them up as high as they'll go easily in the direction of the X yet still rest on the floor. You can also support your arms on pillows if that helps you to get closer to the X position. Bend your knees again and put your feet into standing position. Imagine someone holding your right arm and gently pushing the whole arm in toward your torso, with the arm remaining straight. It will feel like your shoulder blade is moving on the floor toward your spine.

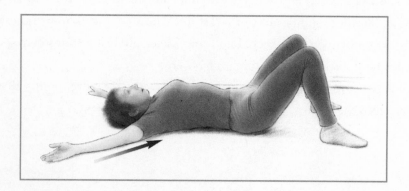

Try that movement several times. See if you can feel the straight arm sliding inward toward your back. Now as you slide your arm, can you try tilting your right leg to the left? Try tilting your leg to the left and sliding the arm a couple of times. Rest.

Try the same sequence on the left side.

Return to the same X position, but now let both knees tilt—once to the right and once to the left. Sense your ribs, your sternum (breastbone), and your neck. What does your head want to do? Do your legs move as one unit, or do they move one leg at a time? Whichever way you were doing it, now try the other way. Rest.

Return to your seated position, leaning back on your hands. Try tilting your legs side to side again. What does it feel like now? What is the action of the chest? Stand up and walk around. As you walk, notice the position of your chest. What is it like now to shift the chest? Is it different somehow?

Take a few minutes to write down your impressions.

TOWARD A NEW YOU

Think of someone you have been avoiding—either speaking to them or calling them. Perhaps it's someone you really admire but feel really shy around. Maybe there's someone who drives you crazy with her constant complaining or a person with whom you've recently disagreed and are feeling uncomfortable with. As you think about speaking to this person, notice your breath. Can you hear the beat of your heart? Make a point of speaking to that person—it could be just one sentence. See if you can maintain an easy breathing pattern as you speak, or if your breath, and even your awareness of your breath, just evaporates the minute you begin to speak!

Exploration Checklist

☐ Play with various positions of the chest, noticing how they affect your walk and emotions.

☐ Try to catch yourself in social interactions throughout the day and see what the chest is doing.

☐ Do the Feldenkrais movement sequence that explores inhibiting movement as you breathe.

☐ Take moments out of your day to notice your breath.

☐ Experiment with placing your hands on various parts of the chest to see what expressions it brings up.

☐ Do "The Real You" Feldenkrais movement sequence, which examines your chest's relationship to the spine.

☐ Try the "Toward a New You" exercise on noticing your breath.

Seven

GETTING TO THE CORE—
THE PELVIS AND YOUR SPONTANEITY

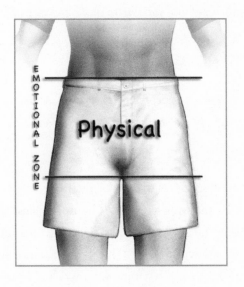

My pelvis is the source of my power.
  How do I see this power?
My pelvis reflects my spontaneity
  and potency. What do people see?
  What do I see?

NICE GIRLS (AND BOYS) DON'T WIGGLE

Western culture frowns on a mobile pelvis. The higher the class, the quieter the pelvis.
Aristocrats favor a body language that indicates lofty thinking, not a reminder that we

have organs and urges. Add to that religious attitudes about sexuality and a cultural distaste regarding natural processes like elimination, and the pelvis becomes an incubator for compulsive behavior that is reflected in movement.

Bill had severe pain in his legs and feet. He had been to orthopedic doctors, neurologists, podiatrists, even psychologists. I asked him to walk across the room. He held his entire torso stiffly and erect, like a soldier. With each step he bent and then locked his knees to heave himself across the room. His pelvis was held rigidly in place with tightly clenched buttocks and a severely arched lower back. After a few lessons, he began to walk with a little movement in his pelvis. He almost fell. "What have you done? I'm wiggling all over the place!" he exclaimed in horror.

"No, you're not," I replied. " It's just that your pelvis is starting to move as you walk."

"Why did you do that?"

It was my turn to be surprised. "Well, your legs move with your pelvis."

"You mean, my pelvis is supposed *to move?"*

Bill was shocked. He spent the next week staring at people as they walked through the supermarket, at doctors' offices, in the street. It was as if he had discovered a new country—and indeed he had.

Several factors have conspired to freeze the contemporary pelvis. As mentioned above, movement of the pelvis has been frowned on by the upper classes. The upper class in general has limited their movements, associating large gestures and broad expression with a class that didn't know how to cover their own feelings ("Keep your hands in your lap, young lady." "It's not polite to point!"). Common people who worked in the fields or did other forms of manual labor needed to engage the pelvis in order to do heavy work. The more refined clerk or businessman relied on his head. Not to mention the fact that much of his time was spent sitting—restricting pelvic motion. Therefore, if one wanted to appear either intelligent or cultured, one restricted pelvic movement.

When Elvis Presley exploded into popular culture, one of his nicknames was "Elvis the Pelvis." As he sang, he used his pelvis in what at the time was considered a provocative fashion. Conservatives and parents were horrified at his gyrations. Somewhere deep in the Western psyche was buried the belief that movement of the pelvis indicates a lascivious nature. Certain religious beliefs stressed the sinfulness of sexual abandon and pleasure, so someone who moved their pelvis while walking was considered sinful. A woman who allows her pelvis to sway is inviting trouble. A man who stands with his pelvis thrust forward (think Mick Jagger) is making a sexual statement. And a man who wiggles is considered a sissy.

Sex and sexuality are big deals. It doesn't matter whether you embrace or try to ignore it, sex affects everything: from the ads on TV, to what you choose to wear, to whom we elect president. The reproductive urge and its affects on all aspects of human functioning cannot be shoved into a corner. In Feldenkrais's book *The Potent Self,* he writes, "Full orgasm accompanied by intense gratification is a physiological necessity for the smooth running of the protective, self-assertive, and recuperative functions. . . . No matter how varied one's life may otherwise be, without the occasional absolute abandonment of the protective and self-assertive habits—as occurs only in frank, spontaneous, and harmonious relationship . . . there always remains an anxious longing for something sensed as an ideal state of peaceful well-being." According to Feldenkrais, the use of the pelvis in standing, walking, and daily life can affect the quality of intimate relationships. If the pelvis is frozen in daily activity, the sexual act is affected as well. How you use your pelvis signals your potency and attractiveness to others. You also make unconscious decisions about potential partners by observing their pelvis ("He seems like a *really* nice guy." "He's a lady killer." "She's a vamp." "She walks like she's got a stick . . .").

DEEP ISSUES

The pelvis can be visualized as a bowl, a container for essential organs, the repository of primal emotions. The relation among these visceral reactions, physiological response, and body language are intimately intertwined. Sudden terror can cause bladder release and even defecation. Profound sexual pleasure resides in the pelvis. We have expressions: "I was so excited, I almost peed in my pants!" "It was a gut-wrenching experience." Because the functions of control and release are major aspects of the functioning of the pelvis, these issues are often reflected in the movement of the pelvis.

It takes tension and effort to inhibit the natural movement of the pelvis. This tension can have many physiological results. Holding the pelvis forces the hip joints to work harder, contributing to joint pain and arthritis. It can also lead to all sorts of back pain—from soreness to spinal stenosis, a painful hardening of the disks, to sciatica. Many times tension in the abdomen contributes to digestive and elimination problems. In coping with stress the pelvis often stiffens and the muscles in the pelvic region begin to grip, as if we are afraid we will "lose our center" if we let go. This counterproductive yet completely understandable reaction then begins a vicious cycle of pain and disease.

Christopher came to me because drugs were no longer helping control his anxiety attacks. He was also in constant pain. He had been taking Vioxx for years until it was recalled. His doctor had no clue as to the cause of his pain, which he described as stiffness in all his joints. When we first started working together he told me about his job worries, his brother's heart problems, and his mother's loneliness since his dad died. When I asked him to lie on the table, he would always want to lie his stomach. If I asked him to take another position, he would oblige but lie there stiff with a fixed expression on his face, as if he was enduring something. If I would ask him if he was okay, he'd say, unconvincingly, "I'm fine, just fine."

As our trust developed, one day he confided that he had been sexually abused when he was a little boy by an uncle that was living in their home. The uncle was only a teenager, but everyone knew him as the family brute. He was violent and temperamental. He would come into Christopher's room late at night, rape him, and then threaten him. He told Christopher that he would kill him if he ever breathed a word of their "playtime." So Christopher had kept his mouth shut for over thirty years.

We began working with movements that explore flexion and extension of the spine, curling into a fetal position, then stretching out to full height. He confessed that the stretching out was very uncomfortable. He told me he suffered from chronic lower intestinal pain and cramping, which he described as gut wrenching. In fact, he had had stomach problems since the time the abuse began. He constantly was overcome with severe pain and nausea, spending "a lot of time with the school nurse." No one was able to find a cause for his problems, and he was diagnosed as a high-strung and nervous child.

As we continued, slowly, within what Christopher considered to be his safety range, the knots in his intestines slowly relaxed. In spite of his intelligence and his years of therapy, Christopher had been unable to teach his body that the world was safe. His body's fear of violation and reprisal had remained locked in his pelvis, preventing him from effective functioning, sexual pleasure, and intimacy. Only by listening to his own movement has he slowly been able to reclaim his own potency.

Deep Knowing

Part 1

Working with metaphor often can help to answer questions we have about parts of ourselves. Choose a time when you have a few minutes for contemplation; you can put on some quiet music or work in silence. Grab something to draw with—crayons, markers, or whatever is available. You can include this exercise in your journal or use a separate sheet of paper. Close your eyes and picture your pelvis as a bowl. What kind of bowl would it be? Plain, fancy, symmetrical, deep, shallow, precious, or utilitarian? Let your imagination play. Now draw the bowl on a piece of paper, then write down the following words—Sex, Elimination, Control, Release, Pleasure, Pain—placing them either inside or outside the bowl. Some words might be big, some might be small. You might find yourself using one word several times, or you might not be able to find a place for other words. Where do these issues reside in you? Which ones carry weight, are the most important? After completing this part, you may wish to stop for the day, or you may wish to continue right away with the next part.

PART 2

After studying where you have placed the words in relation to your bowl, begin to free associate. Ask yourself questions about your choices. Write about why one or the other aspect was more or less important. You can let words spill at random, or you may find yourself writing a story about something from your childhood. You may find yourself listing symptoms of illnesses or pain that you have experienced. Often during workshops, students have encountered resistance at this "art project." In most cases, they've realized hidden attitudes and fears concerning the naming of their pelvis struggles. If you find yourself harrumphing or dismissing the exercise, don't force anything. Let it go, return to it some other time. Or sit and study your attitude. What are you really feeling? Allow yourself to deepen your relationship with this central part of yourself.

PART 3

Go for a walk. As you walk, notice what you feel in this lowest part of your trunk. You may feel nothing at all. We are so accustomed to our habitual way of moving that to discern *how* we move is often difficult at first. You may feel that you are holding your abdomen or, like Bill, your buttocks or lower back are held chronically. As you walk, experiment. (It is best to do this when there are no cars or witnesses about!) Change the way your pelvis moves. Notice how it makes you feel.

PART 4

Go to a public place. If you can, bring your journal. Observe how others use their pelvises and note down your impressions of who you think they are. What would it be like to try on another person's movement? How does their movement, or lack of it, contribute to your idea about their potency? Their sexuality? Their social class?

Note down what you notice about the range, direction, and quality of movement so that you can experiment later with duplicating some of the walks for yourself in private.

PART 5

When you are at home, try some of the walks you observed. Note your reactions— when you are judgmental, when you feel connected to that person's walk, the times you feel frightened, and so on.

TRUCKING, WADDLING, SLITHERING, TRUDGING

While Carla and I were working together to uncover the cause of her sciatic pain, I became concerned that the infections and illnesses she had been fighting for the last six months might be indicative of something more serious. When I watched her walk, it was as if she was carrying a heavy load in her belly. Not full of life like a pregnant woman, but like she was carrying stones that forced her to drag her legs. "Yes, I know what you mean," Carla said. "I've been trudging for months now. I'm literally dragging my ass." We laughed, but I urged her to see a doctor, just in case. It turned out that Carla had uterine cancer. One tumor was so large it was pressing on her organs. We continued meeting until her surgery, and although she still had the weight inside her, her walk changed. As she worked with her personal demons surrounding reproduction, fear, control, rage at her mother, and much more, Carla's walk turned into a flowing earth goddess meander. Her wardrobe changed from sexless T-shirts and sweatpants to flowing batiks, jewelry, and exotic colors. By the time of her surgery she claimed that she had recovered the woman she had suffocated twenty years before. I often see her in town, sauntering and singing. She bought a new car and feels that her liberated pelvis has given her a new life.

The movement of the pelvis affects the quality of the walk and tells a great deal both about the person and where they may be experiencing physical discomfort. There are three possible planes of movement in a well-organized system: rotation, a twisting motion; flexion, an action of the sides of the pelvis going up and down, causing the ribs to bend and straighten; and translation, shifting forward and back/side to side. Ideally these planes smoothly interact to create a pleasing flow, but more often one direction predominates. You can't just look at a pelvic movement and decide what a person is saying. There are women, for example, whose hips sway side to side, but, their backs might be held rigidly and there is no forward/back or up/down. You might say that from the hips a woman like this is a sexy lady, but actually that's the only plane of movement this person has left. She has inhibited the forward and back thrust and the pelvic rotation. A person like this has difficulty getting ahead. Her pelvis has no power. The side-to-side movement slows the walk, making her appear inefficient. Because she is heaving her weight from one leg to the other, she has a precarious sense of balance, which will make her seem even more of a slowpoke. Eventually a walk like this takes its toll in the hip joints, which are bearing the brunt of the weight as the foot strikes.

Bert is a very large man with a jolly demeanor. He loves to eat and drink and often shows up for lessons with crumbs from his candy bars or stains from some treat on his shirt or pants. Bert started coming to see me because his psychotherapist was getting nowhere with him in getting over his self-esteem issues. When I asked Bert to walk across the room, his only plane of movement was lateral flexion, which means that sides of his pelvis moved up and down. His ribs would shorten on one side then the other, tipping his torso left and right. This forced his feet out sideways as well. The impression was of a giant three-year-old boy, still teetering on unsteady legs without access yet to the pelvis. Picture the cliché "jolly" choreography of a musical like Oklahoma where the farmers all bend side to side as they sing, doing an "aw shucks" gesture with the arm and fist. No wonder no one took him seriously! When we began working together he would often fall asleep just when he started to sense how he was moving. One minute he was moving, the next minute he was snoring. He confessed that his parents fought constantly when he was growing up. It was unbearable, so he would go in his room and go to sleep. This unbearable feeling somehow became connected to his body, and he became uncomfortable with any kind of sensation, effectively inhibiting the development of a full range of motion. As we explored how he moved, sometimes I would ask him, "How does your back feel now in comparison with the way it was fifteen minutes ago?" He always began his answer with "It would seem that I am lying flatter" or "One would think that I am more comfortable." He was not able to say, "My back is flatter" or "I feel better."

When we first began working Bert had a dream for starting a new business but no money. I worked with him at a discounted rate. By the time we finished our work, he had given me a "raise" to above my regular fee and his business is now the most successful of its kind. His walk did not transform from a three-year-old boy's to an Olympic athlete. But Bert did discover that he could stand on his own two feet—that he was not going to fall down, and that his body was not something to be ignored or loathed. That discovery shifted his walk enough so that he literally could move ahead with his life.

Having access to all planes of movement in the pelvis does not mean that you need excessive movement. Moving the pelvis too much creates an emphasis that can send a definite signal as well.

Christy's role model growing up was Marilyn Monroe. She perfected the sex kitten voice and began her professional life as a stripper. From there she studied African dance, becoming one of the most successful in her field. No one would accuse her of a frozen pelvis! But she never could find a permanent relationship. Men were attracted to her sexiness, but they left when depth was required. When she came to see me she was in her forties, still beautiful, still sexy, but tired. She had back pain and shoulder pain, and she said she felt like she was falling apart. When she walked her small breasts were thrust forward, as if to belie their size. Her pelvis rolled in a sinewy fashion as her shoulders swayed from side to side. The impression was of someone who was moving in parts—as if she had studied several fifties movie stars and grabbed a slither from one, a shoulder roll from another, a toss of the head from the third. This made her steps quite small. When I asked her to stride, her entire walk changed. It was actually assertive, almost masculine. From years of dance her pelvis knew exactly how to propel her body across the room. It was clear that Christy was hiding her light under a bushel. Her true female power was disguised by this sex-kitten role. I asked her how she felt striding around. She laughed. "Like a man!" As we worked together, Christy found a way to blend her two extremes. With her newfound assertiveness, she realized that she had chosen her various careers in order to serve. She decided that she was free to serve not just men but all people, including herself. She is now in medical school.

The Pelvic Clock

This exercise can serve many purposes. It can provide awareness of how you use your pelvis in movement and can provide new options that will make your walk more fluid and easier. Although this lesson emphasizes awareness of pelvic movement, you will also learn how the pelvis influences and connects with the rest of your skeletal system, which can have the added benefit of reducing tension and pain. And because the movements are not large, you can do variations of this lesson almost anywhere—in a hotel room while traveling, at your desk, at a stoplight. It is best to try it for the first time in a place where you can lie down comfortably on a firm surface. If it is difficult for you to get to the floor, you can do this exercise on a bed.

Begin by walking and noticing your pelvic movement. Which direction is predominant for you? Forward/back translation, rotation, flexion? Some combination? None of the above? Just notice without judgment.

Now lie on your back with your legs stretched long. Notice how much of your back contacts the floor. How does your pelvis touch the floor? Is the weight evenly distributed or does it seem heavier or lighter on one side? Or perhaps you are pressing on the tailbone more than the top of the sacrum. Just notice.

Bend your knees and put your feet at a comfortable distance from each other so that you don't need to use a lot of tension to hold your legs up. Imagine a clock underneath your pelvis, as if your pelvis was lying on the face of a clock. Imagine that

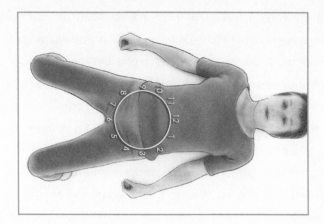

noon on the clock is under the top of your pelvis, where your belt would be. Six o'clock is at the tip of the tailbone. That would place three o'clock under the left side of the pelvis and nine o'clock under the right. Just take a moment to see that in your mind's eye.

Begin to tilt your pelvis so that you are pressing your pelvis on noon. In other words, your tailbone comes up a bit in the air and your belt line presses down. Then return to neutral. Try that movement several times. As you tilt your pelvis, allow your attention to travel. How do you do this movement? Often the answer is "I don't know!"

I once asked this question of an eighty-year-old client who had never paid attention to her body's movement in spite of constant pain. She looked at me in amazement and burst out, "How do I move it? Sheer will!"

After tilting several times, rest. You can rest with your legs stretched out or leave them bent.

If your legs are long, bend them again and place your feet on the floor as before. Begin tilting the opposite way, pressing onto six o'clock several times. As you do this movement, notice if you feel any movement in your head. Is this direction easier or more difficult for you? Are your feet doing anything?

Begin tilting your pelvis back and forth between six and twelve. Can you feel your head moving now? As you tilt your pelvis, it pushes and pulls your spine. This in turn affects the head, so that in effect you have a little clock under your head as well. Continue moving up and down and see if you can increase the speed. It doesn't have to be a big movement; in fact let it get smaller as it gets faster, so that you just start to jiggle up and down. Feel your head moving with your pelvis.

Rest. As you're resting, clarify your image of the rest of the clock. Try to see clearly where on your pelvis the other numbers will fall.

When you feel ready, bend your knees again and slowly begin moving your pelvis around the clock. There are many ways to do this—you can do a few numbers at a time, exploring the upper arc, the lower arc, or the sides in a half circle, or you can start going slowly around the whole clock. Whichever way you decide to explore, take your time to notice details about the various hours. Are there numbers that are easier to touch than others? Are you making a smooth circle, or are there sections where you cut a straight line? Can you move your head in concert with your pelvis, circling around a little head clock? What do your feet do? Your knees? Do you feel anything in your back against the floor? Make sure you take time to rest whenever you feel like you are beginning to strain. After doing this several times, rest, and then resume the movement, eventually making circles both clockwise and counterclockwise.

You can stop here, or if you'd like a further investigation, try moving your pelvis in one direction and your head in the opposite direction. Let it be fun.

For a sitting variation, you can place the clock underneath your seat on your chair. Three and nine o'clock remain virtually the same. Now noon and six o'clock become the result of rounding your back and curling your tailbone under (noon) and arching your low back slightly so that your pubis comes forward (six). You still can circle in both directions, and you also can move your head, which is very interesting. But don't do this while driving!

When you are finished, come to standing and take a walk around. See if your experience of locomotion has changed. What do you feel in your pelvis?

HOLDING BACK/RELEASING YOUR PERSONAL POWER

Potency and *potential* come from the same root word: *potentia.* Impotence, frigidity, compulsion, all reside in a frozen pelvis. Freeing the pelvis can be both exhilarating and terrifying. It means you're free to move ahead. Or sideways. You can charge ahead or get out of the way, sometimes your own way. How does this affect creativity, personal freedom, and productivity?

> *Mark approached me after a class where I had taught the Pelvic Clock lesson, his eyes cast down. "That lesson was a problem for me," he muttered. "It is not good to awaken those feelings. I've been trying to forget about sex, to accept that I'll never have sex again. As I was doing the movements, I could feel my sexuality rising up. I can't allow it to take over."*
>
> *"Why not?" I asked.*
>
> *He smiled bitterly. "I guess you didn't notice that I'm seventy-three years old. I haven't been with a woman since my divorce eighteen years ago. I have to accept that I'm going to spend the rest of my life alone."*
>
> *"Why?"*
>
> *He scoffed. "At my age? With this body? Who'd want me?" He hastened away, already returning to his military march, his heels hitting the ground sharply, his arms stiff by his sides. If I were a woman I'd think twice about potential romance. His every move said "Stay away! I am angry and asexual!"*

Your pelvis links you with a source of power, spontaneity, and freedom in yourself. It contains your body's center of gravity. This center has many names in different cultures, many of which are synonyms in their language for *spirit* or *power: tai-tien* or *dantian* in Chinese, *hara* in Japanese, *kath* in Arabic, *spiritus* in Latin, *ruach* in Hebrew. According to noted psychologist and teacher Karlfried Graf Durckheim in his book *Hara: The Vital Center of Man,* "The hara designates the part of the lower abdomen and pelvis region near the genital organs. It is an area located one and a half inches below the navel and one and a half inches inward toward the spine. This point also happens to be the body's central axis (center of gravity/balancing point). The word *hara* literally translates to *belly*." In yogic tradition, the pelvis houses the first and second chakras, both involved in the functions of control, release, creativity, and support.

A centered or grounded person is someone you can rely on to be able react appropriately in any given situation. Most martial arts stress this relationship with the pelvis. Morihei Ueshiba, the founder of aikido, was under five feet tall, yet he was considered Japan's finest martial artist and was never defeated. Even in his eighties, frail and ill, he merely had to turn his pelvis toward his attacker and the latter would fly across the room and land with a crash. Someone who walks with the pelvis as their center of gravity has greater control of the legs, can turn more quickly, and gives the impression of strength and agility. However, many people place their center of gravity on other parts. Culturally we have been encouraged to place our center in the chest or the head, which has a two-fold effect. The nineteenth- and early-twentieth-century ideal posture was standing tall with the chest out. This posture was considered noble and stouthearted. It also effectively freezes the pelvis. The Victorian and puritanical belief system encouraged both sexual repression and the repression of movement in the pelvis.

Someone whose head leads is often thought of as a lofty thinker, or perhaps the person fancies herself as such. For the head to rule, there is a constant tugging on the neck, creating tension from the shoulders down. This person is always in danger of falling—either because her head is in the clouds or because her head is literally dragging her body around. Once again, pelvic movement is constrained, and an observer will note that this person does not live in the passions.

Marilyn is a physicist, brilliant and funny, who walks without moving any part of her trunk, her arms held stiffly, as if her body hung from her head. "I'm sorry," she once said. "I just don't get what you mean by a center of gravity. Of course my pelvis is my center of gravity! It's heavy and it's in the middle of my body! According to the laws of physics, it has to be in the center. My head is at the top!" While Marilyn is full of joie de vivre, she has created many physical limitations for herself, with consequent discomfort because her only freely moving part is her neck. I explained that center of gravity is not just a physical location, but the place from which one chooses to initiate movement. From the point of view of physics, Marilyn suddenly saw that she had been perceiving her body as a head that commands a large appendage, like a driver of a large machine.

With both of the above postural choices, the inhibition of the pelvis also may reflect various forms of compulsive behavior that are not always visible upon first glance. In *The Potent Self* Feldenkrais wrote, "In any particular case of impotence, including sexual impotence and frigidity, there is a lack of motility of the pelvis and defective abdominal tone due to personal experience, as opposed to biological inheritance."

Sometimes people who place their center of gravity in other parts of the skeleton can distort their relationship to sex. For example, in the case of the chest centered, think obsessive romantics and stalkers. Clerics and professors often assume a head-centered posture, which sometimes suggests repressed drives of the sort that have resulted in church- and academic-based sex scandals in recent years.

That is not to say that every person who disengages from the pelvis is a sexual predator; it is merely one facet of a multidimensional portrait. People have many reasons for choosing to freeze the pelvis, as we've seen in the many previous examples.

Finding Your Center

What is your true center of gravity? It's not just about what leads or is more predominantly forward. You can try the following experiment alone or with a friend. Intentionally begin to walk with your pelvis as your center of gravity, meaning you generate your movement from the pelvic region. If this is difficult to achieve, you can exaggerate the feeling by slightly bending your knees, which has the effect of bringing the attention to your center. Play with letting the pelvis lead, move, freeze, and go backward. Then try bringing your focus to your chest. You can lead with the chest, but also notice what happens when you intentionally decide that your chest is the center of you. A person actually could have a collapsed chest and still make that their center if all of their manifestations came from a place of self pity and insecurity, for example. Then try walking with your head as your center of gravity. Notice which of these centers feels like home to you. It's possible that you feel comfortable in more than one—we may switch centers depending on the situation we are in. With each of these experiments, ask yourself the following questions:

1. How would this person respond to change and surprise?
2. What do I feel in my spine and pelvis when this part leads?
3. Do I tense up anywhere when I use this part of myself?
4. What directions are available for rapid movement (turning, reversing, jumping)?
5. What happens if I have to run like this?

Take some time to record your observations. Now that you've finished this chapter, revisit your pelvic bowl drawing and list of words. Is there any new information available for you?

TOWARD A NEW YOU

Bringing your awareness to your pelvis as you go through life can change the way you deal with any given situation. Here are some suggestions to help you shift a situation by changing your center of gravity.

• Whether you are initiating a call or answering the phone, notice your lower back and how it connects to the pelvis. Often the pelvis freezes and tension starts to mount in the chest and the head. If you can stand and feel the bowl of the pelvis as you speak, you may find the phone conversation less stressful.

• When speaking to someone you find attractive, take note of your pelvis and how your arms and legs are relating to it. Do you feel mobile and free? Have you turned your pelvis slightly away or toward them? One hip cocked? Play with small, subtle changes in your positioning and notice what happens in the conversation.

- As you are walking, intentionally change the way your pelvis moves. You don't have to do this in public, although it can be fun and very revealing if you do. Notice the power of your gait and your attitude. If possible, steal a glimpse of yourself in a store window as you stride past. Who do you see?

Exploration Checklist

- ☐ Explore the concept of your pelvis as a bowl via your drawing and placement of words.
- ☐ Try the "Deep Knowing" exercise—looking at your questions surrounding functions in the pelvis.
- ☐ Give yourself the time to try the Pelvic Clock exercise.
- ☐ Experiment with changing your center of gravity.
- ☐ Record your observations.
- ☐ Play with the suggestions in "Toward a New You."

Eight

IT'S ALL IN YOUR HEAD

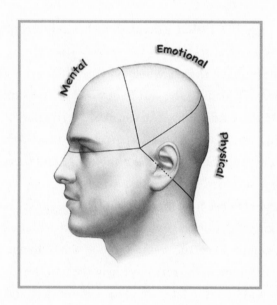

How I carry my head tells the world my attitude. Do I know where my head is?

The placement of my head affects my balance and direction. Where am I going and how am I getting there?

IT'S WHAT'S INSIDE THAT COUNTS

Years ago there was a V8 commercial that showed someone sipping a drink. All of a sudden he claps his hand to his forehead and says, "I could have had a V8!" The message was "Don't forget this alternative juice is available." But the expression also became a line people use when they've forgotten something and feel a need to slap their palm comically on their foreheads.

Think of all the gestures people use in relation to the head—scratching the temples or the top, resting chin in hand, rubbing mouth, chin, nose, cheeks, or the back of the neck. Think of the famous Rodin sculpture the *Thinker,* sitting supporting his head with his fist. Do all of these gestures have a physiological basis? It's possible that they do.

Oh Boy!

As you can see in the illustration on page 109, Delsarte divided the head into zones based on the trinity.

We now know that even though the brain works as a whole system, different areas of the brain regulate various functions. Touching the different areas of the skull seems to reflect emotions connected to these functions. You can easily verify the different qualities of the head by bringing your hand to various parts of the head—the forehead, the mid brain, the back of the skull. Each time you bring your hand there, use an expression related to memory, such as "Oh boy, that was some party last night!" Delsarte suggested using "I can't believe how much I drank last night!" You also can simply try "What was I thinking?" Notice if your face takes a particular expression. Does your head change position? Does the sound of your voice change? There are myriad ways of discerning meaning in the relationship of the hands to the head and face. As we explore the face and hands in later chapters, your understanding of the various relationships and connections will deepen. Meanwhile, feel free to observe and take notes on the variety of gestures you discover while people watching or by studying your own choices.

WHERE'S YOUR HEAD?

The class members all lowered their heads and began to walk around the room. "Depressed," stated one. "Nearsighted," announced another. "Not very healthy," averred a third. "Reminds me of my childhood," said Al. When we were seated, he continued, "When I was young I always looked down at the floor. My father was always yelling, 'Straighten up! Pick up your head!' but I couldn't." Al now walks with his head jutting forward and his chest sunk deeply down, with a little shuffle. I asked Al if he remembers what it was like to straighten up at his father's commands. "I couldn't do it—I would try, but I just couldn't."

"You mean your spine was fused or something like that?"

"No. I couldn't see where I was going."

"Were you nearsighted?"

"Yes, but that's not it. It, it just didn't feel safe. If I looked up, there was too much to see."

In theater the head's position often defines a character. Thrust forward it signifies aggression. When forward and slightly down, a quality of shyness or weariness creeps into the portrayal. In just these two examples you can see how the physiological and psychological begin to relate. The head thrust forward takes the spine out of balance. You must keep moving forward or you'll fall down. To compensate, you have to hunch and engage your shoulders, grip the trapezius and sternocleidomastoid muscles (the ropelike muscles on the side of the neck), and sometimes even tense your jaw. With that level of tension, no wonder a person feels aggressive! With the head forward and little down, the person's skeleton is losing the battle with gravity. The aggression has been thwarted. The upper spine needs to round a bit to keep the head from falling farther and compromising balance. The eyes need to peer upward. As with hunched shoulders, it is difficult to turn the head quickly from side to side, making the person vulnerable to anything coming from the side. And with the spine all rounded, there isn't enough freedom for a quick directional change. This is a very insecure feeling, not to mention extremely tiring. Thus the person is both physically and psychologically insecure and weary.

The stress of holding the head up in these orientations ultimately affects the person's health in many ways. The tension in the neck muscles often leads to severe headaches. Sometimes when the head is held forward the jaw muscles become engaged, leading to TMJ (temporomandibular joint disorder), a common syndrome in which the jaw is so tense that those afflicted have been known to break their teeth. A lifetime of carrying the head forward creates many compensatory habits that can ultimately lead to dowager's hump, a kind of humped rounding at the vertebrae on the top of the shoulder girdle. Vision problems are also created by the straining and narrow focus.

There are ergonomic and cultural factors at work here as well. A primary change in the use of our skeletons has taken place in the last century. Previously most people worked outdoors or engaged in other physical activities. With the industrial age came automation and office jobs that required long periods of either standing in place or sitting down. The skeleton is designed for movement. Standing or sitting for a long time can produce stress on the skeleton, creating a struggle for balance. When you sit a long time, for example, the lower back can start to feel tight if the head-pelvis relationship is not comfortable and supported. You want to slouch, round over, and the head starts to move downward. Add to that all the different demands for looking straight forward in a focused fashion: driving a car, staring at a computer screen, assembling a product for hours on end. This affects both the freedom of the head and the functioning of the eyes. In some so-called undeveloped nations, people often have to walk from place to place, often carrying their luggage on their heads. If the head and pelvis are not connected by an integrated spine, carrying a weight becomes uncomfortable very quickly. But with everything organized the head easily can sustain weights that are too much for just the arms.

When you see a person with her head hanging down and her back rounded, you get the impression of someone who is not physically active, vital, or strong. And often people come to me for lessons because both their physical and emotional lives have been affected by the postural demands of their jobs. They feel less alive and less energetic as a result of hours of sitting or working at the computer. On the opposite side of the coin, a person who walks with head back or chin up conveys an attitude of retreat, which can be interpreted as anything from fear to arrogance (nose in the air, stuck up, and so on). In terms of Delsarte's zones, bringing the head back indicates the mind retreating from the object or person, and therefore not wanting to engage intellectually. In both cases the posture and the attitude become a kind of vicious circle—one habit reinforcing the other, the physical affecting the emotional, and vice versa.

It is important, however, to remember to look at the person as a whole. Too often we are taken by one aspect of a person's body language and miss subtle cues that can affect our interactions. Al, who I used in the previous example, appears weak and physically challenged. Yet he is afraid of countless things, from running out of money to whether he'll get back home in time to walk his dogs. He is, nevertheless, also a very opinionated and strong-minded person, and therefore his anger sometimes overpowers his fears and he lashes out unexpectedly. In some ways he uses his weak appearance to manipulate others to get what he needs. Al has bought into his identity as a wimp and uses that mask as a weapon. The payoff for his learning to walk freely and upright would be a complete change in his self-image, something he is not willing to do.

Playing with Your Head

Studying where you habitually carry your head can yield tremendous insights on your attitudes—both physical and emotional. In the exercises in Chapter 2 you may have noticed the position of your head in relation to your plumb line. Was it in front, behind, or right in the center? Was it to the right or the left? Feel free to check again right now. Without trying to correct your head's position, begin walking around, feeling what your relation to your head's position is now. We often are so accustomed to our holding patterns that we don't feel anything at all. Whatever pattern you noticed—either in the mirror or in your walk—intentionally exaggerate it. In other words, if you noticed that your head is slightly forward, extend it a bit more. Or if your head is slightly to the left or right, let it go farther. Keep walking around and see where you feel the pull on your skeletal organization. Now bring it back to neutral.

Play for a while with the different positions of the head. See what it feels like to walk with your head back or up slightly. Notice how it affects the rest of your body and your emotions. Nothing happens in isolation. One person will bring the head back and suddenly the chest puffs out, giving an impression of self-importance. Another will bring the head back and suddenly the eyes widen in an expression of terror. By doing this simple exercise you may discover that you have a preferred repertoire of emotions. Or you may discover that you have no idea at all what your body conveys. Both of these are important observations. Give yourself time to record your impressions—even if your impression is that you felt nothing.

Sometimes people say they feel like they have a stiff neck. While this is a valid observation, according to Delsarte's terminology it is a condition, not a sentiment. It is a physical state, not an emotion. You want to go further to see if a sentiment exists that is the cause or the result of the observed condition.

Putting Your Head in Its Place ⟩

Find a comfortable seated posture, either in a straight-backed chair with your feet on the floor and your back away from the chair back, or sitting cross-legged on the floor. Notice how it feels to sit. Where is your head right now? Begin a movement of lowering your head and raising it. Repeat this movement several times, moving slowly, listening to the quality of your movement. Does your head go straight up and down, or does it favor going to the right or left a bit? Don't worry if you can't tell. As you continue to lower and raise your head, what do you feel in your chest and back? Do they remain still or is there movement? When do you inhale? When do you exhale? Pause a moment. If you are sitting on the floor, you can lie down. If you are in a chair, just sit back and relax a moment.

Now return to your working position. Continue lowering and raising your head, but this time intentionally exhale as you lower your head and inhale as you raise it. You may notice that your back rounds a bit as you exhale and lower your head. Can you exaggerate that movement a little, letting your ribs soften and your chest move downward as you exhale, and then letting your spine stretch and your chest expand as you look upward? As you do this movement, can you feel how your head sits on top of the spine? As you continue moving in this way, let your attention travel farther down your body. Do you feel anything in your pelvis—movement, stillness, effort, ease? Just observe. Now take another rest.

Return to your working position. This time as you raise and lower your head, moving your chest, sensing your breath, can you include some movement in the pelvis? Remember the movement of the pelvis in Chapter 7 and how it connected to the head. Here you are exploring it from the other orientation. As you lower your head, try letting your pelvis slump back. Feel as if you are trying to touch the back of the chair or the wall with the small of your back. At the same time press your abdomen against your spine. You're not tightening your belly; you're just flattening it into yourself. Then, as you raise your head, tilt your pelvis forward, push your belly out, and let your lower back arch a little. It is okay to stick your belly out. There is a whole relationship of muscles in your front and back that is changed when you expand and contract your belly. If we understood this relationship better, we'd have fewer flabby stomach issues and fewer abdominal problems.

When you go out, do some people watching. Sit yourself down at a café or on a bench at the mall and watch the people walking by. Notice the position of their heads. Notice the judgments and thoughts that move through your mind as you observe them ("That person sure is in a hurry," "Look at that silly girl," and so on). What does the carriage of the head have to do with how you observe them? As you sit and observe, play with your own head's position. Do you look at people differently when your head is leaning forward eagerly? What do your eyes do if you pull your head back?

TALKING HEAD

Check yourself out the next time you see a puppy. Or when someone passes a cute baby into your arms. Chances are your head will tilt a little to the side as you regard the sweetie pie. Along with your postural choices, the head takes certain attitudes in conversations and relationships. When combined with the eyes, eyebrows, and mouth, the head can express myriad emotions.

Whether you are a Darwinist (and Darwin was an avid animal watcher!) or you believe all creatures are linked through some intelligent design, there is no question that many of our expressions are similar to those of animals. The attitudes of the head are an especially wonderful place to remember our relationship with our fellow creatures.

The basic attitudes of the head do not include rotation or combining directions, but they are a good place to begin. Try taking each of these positions and see what they evoke. You'll notice that there is a difference in the emotion depending on where your eyes are looking—in the center, sideways, down, and so on. Each position of the eyes can evoke a different emotional response and is key to interpreting many postures correctly. I will mention a few noteworthy eye-head relationships in Chapter 9, but for now just try out the different positions of the head while moving your eyes into different positions. You'll see that each eye position evokes a different response. Take some notes about what effects the different eye directions have.

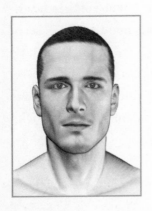

1. The head is sitting straight on the spine.
   This is as close to neutral as we get.

2. The head is tilted.
   According to Delsarte, when we tilt toward something it means we are interested in that object. Think of how you might regard the cup of coffee on your desk as you con-

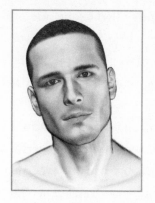

template another sip. When you tilt away, you are distancing your mind from the object. When the eyes are centered, you might be trying to clear something from your head. But try tilting your head away from a friend while keeping your eyes on him. It evokes a feeling of suspicion—"Oh, really?" The combination of the head retreating and the sideways look tells the other "I don't trust you." It's as if the brain is looking askance.

Often when you are facing someone you will find yourself tilting your head for no apparent reason, while still looking directly at them. Just as tilting toward the coffee cup means you're enjoying the brew, tilting our heads this way lets people know we are on their side. Both Delsarte and Susana Bloch call this a position that evokes tenderness. If you look at paintings of certain saints you will see their heads tilted, and, as mentioned earlier, often the whole spine is curved as a result. Artists have used the curve of the spine to signify receptiveness for centuries. In an attempt not to seem direct and confrontational, many women have a tendency to tilt their heads, especially when talking to men. Dogs take this position when they are listening and interested, and their owners interpret it as a kind of affectionate regard. An image used for Edison's early records shows a dog tilting his head toward a Victrola with the slogan "His master's voice."

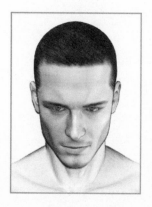

3. The head sinks down the center.

Thinking and concentration, as well as humility or sadness, can be indicated by a lowered head, depending on how the rest of the body responds. A child takes this posture when being scolded, and a professor may take this position while pondering. A panhandler might assume this position, but watch what his or her eyes are doing . . .

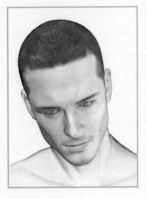

4. The head is lowered and then slightly tilted to one side.

Think of the way you look down at a baby in your arms or of some of the pictures of the Virgin Mary holding the Baby Jesus. It combines tenderness with deep contemplation, what Delsarte called tender adoration.

The sentiment changes entirely, however, when the head is tilted away from someone. I often encountered this powerful gesture when I first set foot in an inner-city school. "Who do you think you are?" it says. "I don't trust you—you are here to take advantage of me, or to flaunt your good fortune." Envy and suspicion are both masks for fear. The fear reaction often involves a retreating motion of the head—tilting the head hides the deeper expression.

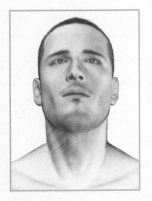

5. The head is thrown straight back between the shoulders.

This position can express a range of emotions, from "Wahoo!" to "Oh my God, I beg you," depending on the rest of the body, especially the face and arms. It can bring the entire skeleton into extension, which means an arching position. Extension excites the nervous system and expands the solar plexus. Therefore it can be Snoopy doing his happy dance, or it can be the shock and grief depicted in Picasso's *Guernica*. In both cases the head thrown back indicates a wish to connect with a higher source—you are filled with life. If done with the spine rounded, it signifies surrender to something greater. It has been described as the manifestation of *agape,* which is a Greek word for unconditional love.

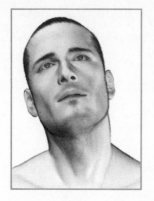

6. The head is back and tilted.

You've seen your dog do this! His head is up and tilted back, staring at you in adoration. It is the pose of the famous statue of Saint Teresa being visited by an angel and pierced by the dart of divine love.

Now change your angle and eyes slightly so that your head is tilted away from the person you are regarding. "Harrumph!" Haughtiness, arrogance, perhaps a bit of distrust are evoked when you withdraw your head and tilt your chin up away from someone or something. It can range from shock to superiority depending again on the gesture's relation to the body.

I Don't Know

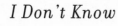

This exercise is really fun to do with a friend, but you can also do it in a mirror. Try repeating the words "I don't know." Each time you say it, choose a different attitude of the head. Notice if the attitude affects the way you say the words, how the rest of you follows. What do your hands want to do? Does the expression on your face change? The tone of your voice? Take note if any seem familiar.

TOWARD A NEW YOU

Pick a few times during the day when you are with others and notice what their heads are doing, and what *your* head likes to do. Do you tend to look at your feet when talking to a superior? Do you tilt your head as you listen? If you notice your head taking a position, intentionally stay in that position for a few moments. See if any feelings come up. Then intentionally change it.

Take the time to record what you notice—were they feelings, thoughts, or sensations? Did you notice physical discomforts? Unexamined attitudes? Unexpressed fears? Your head is a powerful teacher, but only if you pay attention.

Exploration Checklist

- ☐ Return to the plumb line exercise from Chapter 2 and notice how you carry your head.
- ☐ Experiment with the movement lesson "Putting Your Head in Its Place."
- ☐ Try the nine attitudes of the head and note down your responses to the various positions.
- ☐ Go people watching. Notice how people carry their heads and your responses to them.
- ☐ Try the "I Don't Know" exercise.
- ☐ In "Toward a New You," observe how you and others use the head in conversation. How does your head position relate to feeling, sensation, and thought? Take time to write down your observations.

Nine

FACE IT

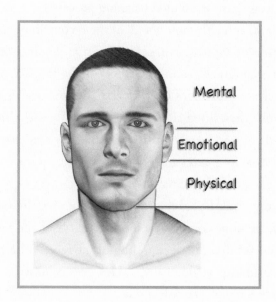

My face masks and reveals my thoughts.
What am I revealing? What am
I hiding?
My face tells the story of my life. What
is my story and how do I feel about it?

There is a saying often attributed to Abraham Lincoln that you can't do anything about the face you were born with, but your face after forty is all your fault. From the moment we are born we are arranging our faces—those first grimaces an infant makes are an attempt to imitate the facial expressions he is seeing on Mom. Within nine minutes of birth infants prefer a face pattern to an abstract or scrambled pattern.

My parents came to visit me one summer after having moved to a distant state. I hadn't seen them in over a year. One day my father decided to join me in weeding the garden. At one point we both reached for the same tool. He screwed up his face in a clownish scowl of determination and anger. I let the tool go in shock. That was my face! It was one of my characteristic expressions—I used it often with my clown characters when they were angry or struggling. I even had pictures of myself using that expression. In that moment I realized that I really didn't know what was essentially me and what I had unconsciously picked up from my parents. While the jury is still out in the nature versus nurture debate (how much of our behavior is learned and how much is genetic?), all agree that imitation is a huge part of a child's learning process.

There are forty-four muscles in the face, and although not all of them contribute to every facial expression, the various nuances of expression are the subject of volumes of research and books beyond Paul Ekman's oeuvre. Certainly what occurs on the face is reflected in the rest of the self. In fact, certain muscles of the face actually seem to trigger different postures. Just try keeping your chest lifted and your step sprightly with the corners of your mouth turned down and your eyebrows knitted together. By studying your own face with its habits and its potential for expression, you can begin to approach the immense learning contained in this one part of the anatomy.

Most of us don't make large expressions, and the subtleness of a drooping eyelid or a slightly flared nostril is rarely noticed, let alone consciously interpreted. And yet we have countless expressions that reflect our intuitive understanding of the face. "There was something in his eyes," "Her lip curled up sardonically," "Her eyes crinkled in amusement," and "His nostrils flared menacingly" are only a few.

Our facial expressions can change like clouds drifting and shifting across the sky, hundreds of tiny expressions responding to every single impression that is being taken in. And at the same time the face also reflects the character of a person, the inner world that she inhabits. The habitual way a person presents herself—her mask, so to speak, tells us if she is moody, aggressive, timid, compassionate, or jolly by nature. And then, to add another layer, what you are seeing may be an actual mask, concealing vulnerable or defensive postures. For example, a perpetually scowling person may be projecting anger in order to disguise fear or deep grief.

As you dive into the following study of the face, remember that you don't have to master this knowledge all at once. That would be like trying to learn how to play Rachmaninoff at your first piano lesson. The human face, indeed the entire organism, is like a complex and marvelous instrument that must be studied and practiced in order for it to yield its wonders. Everything in the face affects the entire self, just like all the other parts. But the face itself has so many parts that one needs to approach it like a body onto itself.

The Mask

In the movie *The Mask* Jim Carrey portrays a loser who happens upon a magical mask of the Norse trickster god Loki, which transforms him into a wild, irresistible prankster. The struggle between the two selves provides the comedy. A mask concealing or revealing the inner self is perhaps one of our most ancient devices. The donning of masks of animals, gods, and other forces was once ritual in almost every ancient religion. As theater moved from the sacred to the secular, the mask became a psychological tool, exaggerating aspects of human expression to denote a particular quality.

Take a look at your face in a mirror. Keeping as neutral an expression as possible, notice where lines have formed. If you are too young to have wrinkles, you can still see small lines where habitual expressions leave their mark. I recently ran into an acquaintance and her five-month-old daughter. As the child studied me, she scowled so profoundly that the forehead created a characteristic set of wrinkles that Darwin called the "grief expression." I was utterly taken aback and wondered what I could have done to deserve this expression. The mother laughed. "She's been doing that since she was born. Like her grandfather's expression." When the child relaxed her face, you could see that lines were already beginning to create a very specific little person who was learning an interesting habit from her grandfather.

As you study the lines, can you imagine the expressions that created them? It may be hard to believe Lincoln's statement, yet each of us has created a mask based on our habitual responses to life. Now smile. As your mouth moves, notice your cheeks, your eyes, even your nose. Let your smile turn into a frown. Which of these expressions is easier for you?

Enter this exploration with a spirit of play and experimentation. You may find that this work inspires you to explore the musculature more deeply through the work of Ekman and others.

I Forgot!

This exercise is more fun with a friend, but you can certainly do it in the mirror as well. Using the phrase "I forgot!" bring your hand to various parts of your face. Notice the emotions and expression that come up when you slap your hand to your forehead as opposed to covering your mouth. How does it feel when you put your hand on your cheek? Notice when you choose to use the back (emotional) as opposed to the front (physical) side of your hand. Does it feel different on your face? Feel free to vary what you say—expressions can include "What was I thinking?," "Oh no!," or one that you make up. Notice how each location of the face elicits a different aspect of expression. This is the beginning of exploring the zones of the face.

LAUGHING, TALKING, EATING, AND KISSING

In the myth of Persephone, Persephone's mother, Demeter, entreated the gods to return her daughter, who had been captured by Pluto, Lord of the Underworld. As a result of her imprisonment in Hades, the world was cast in a perpetual winter. The gods agreed to Persephone's return provided she had not eaten any food while in Hades. Thereupon Pluto quickly offered her a pomegranate. Persephone had already eaten three seeds when she heard the news of her release. She immediately dropped the pomegranate to the ground, but because she had eaten the three seeds she had to return to Hades for three months each year, and this became what we know as winter.

Sleeping Beauty was awakened by . . . a kiss.

The mouth, lips, and tongue take in nourishment, they intimately connect us through kissing, and they communicate our needs through talking. One of the first movements of an infant is a sucking motion for breast-feeding that metamorphoses into the pucker of the kiss as we mature. The infant expresses dissatisfaction and discomfort through screaming, which becomes refined into language.

When we speak of someone thin lipped compared to someone with full, sensuous lips, we are assuming this person's potential sexuality by the quality of the mouth. Someone with no chin can be considered weak, whereas Dudley Do-Right has a large, square chin, a caricature of noble masculinity. However, the same jutting chin, depending on where it points, also could indicate prudishness and coldness, while the weak chin can reflect receptiveness, even sensuality. While some of our facial features are inherited, what you do with them is what tells the story. Are the thin lips patrician or puritanical? Are the full lips inviting or pouty and petulant? Is the jaw firm with resolve or shut tight against intruders? Is it relaxed and responsive or slack-jawed?

Delsarte placed the mouth in the physical zone, so the mouth, chin, and jaw often reflect what is happening in the pelvis. In fact, Feldenkrais called the jaw "the little pelvis." It seems that a tight jaw and a tight pelvis are related!

TMJ and lower back pain often are found together. Herpes appears both on the mouth and on the genitals. And just as the pelvic region regulates elimination, the mouth receives nutrition. These openings, or sphincters, in the body are powerful muscles that govern survival itself.

There are many hypotheses on the reasons behind some of our mouth's expressions. A smile is an expression of satiety. When you are smiling you are not in the position to suck; therefore you are no longer hungry. Some people say that babies have a smiling expression on their faces when they are full and about to pass gas. When they see how pleased their parents/caretakers are, they intentionally repeat this smile. Darwin, however, upon careful observation, noted that babies begin a real smile at about forty-five days. This smile eventually grows into little sounds that become laughter. He therefore suggested that a smile is either the beginning of laughter or suppressed laughter, laughter being the ultimate expression of joy. He quoted a four-year-old child's definition of joy: "It is laughing, talking, and kissing"—all things done with the mouth.

Darwin also observed that the mouths of dogs are wide open when they are uncontrollably happy and are jumping around and barking. In contrast, when they are feeling aggressive the teeth are bared, with an extra curling of the lip to reveal the canines—a snarl. He observed that in certain situations the revealing of the canine only occurs on the side that is facing the threatening animal. When we sneer in contempt, we raise one side of the lip—not enough to reveal the canines, but just enough to communicate our aggressive opinion. And moments of rage often produce the same snarl as a dog.

Among the guests at a dinner party I attended recently was an attractive middle-aged woman known for her philanthropy. Extremely thin (you can never be too rich or too thin) and elegantly dressed, she was surrounded by "friends." As she regaled them with a story, her lips periodically would raise, the two upper corners of her mouth lifting more than the center, revealing her canines. Even as she engaged in social repartee, her rage and resentment at something—her life?, the party?, other people's desire for her money?—sent everyone a very mixed message of contempt and aggression.

Read My Lips

There are nine sets of muscles that govern the movement of the mouth, and at least nine expressions for each set. Multiply this into combinations of muscles and you have a myriad of possibilities. And when you add the rest of the face, you can begin to understand the vastness of our expressive range. Most of our expressions are minute and often barely discernable, but by studying your own mouth you can begin to see how the mouth conveys emotions. The following are nine basic expressions to try in front of the mirror.

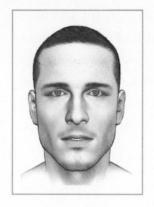
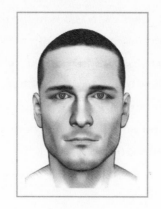
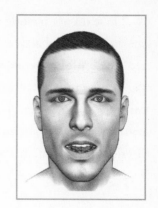
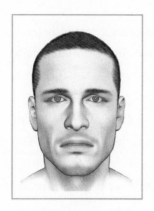
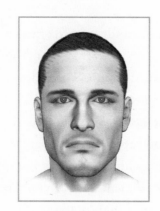
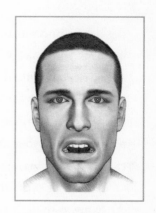
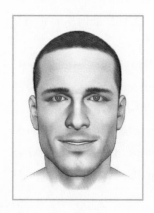
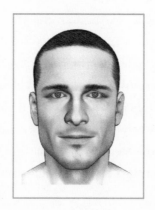
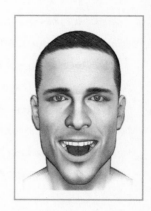

These do not include many other expressions in the mouth's repertoire, such as the snarls mentioned above. As you move your mouth, notice which of these expressions are "you." Which seem difficult to make? How do you feel about the person you are looking at? Try to sense whether the various expressions have any effect on the rest of your carriage. Notice what happens in your abdomen when you frown, for example. Does your chest change slightly as you smile? Like every other part of the body, the expressions in the lips interact with all the other parts.

Lip (and Jaw) Service ⁀

Besides communicating your attitude toward others, your mouth is constantly feeding back information to the rest of your system. Your posture and emotional state are intricately linked with your mouth. The following movement experiment can help you begin to sense the part your mouth plays.

First, go to a mirror and take a look at your face. Notice the sense of relaxation or tension around your mouth and eyes. You may want to sense your posture as well. You can do the following sequence either lying down or sitting.

Close your eyes for a few moments and let your awareness travel to your mouth. Are your teeth tightly together or slightly apart? How do your lips feel? Are the corners of your mouth down, up, or neutral? Don't worry if you can't tell; this kind of attention takes practice. The following movement experiment will help you notice more about your mouth.

First, try to let your lower jaw open slightly a few times. You can let it open on its own, or you can place your hands gently on your chin and pull it open and shut, very slowly, a few times. What does it feel like to open your mouth? Many people have spent a lifetime swallowing their words, repressed from childhood or perhaps frustrated from not being heard. Opening the mouth in this way can be an unnerving experience. Respect your comfort level and make sure to do the exercise slowly. If you do it quickly, you will feel nothing, except perhaps more tension. Notice what you feel in the back of your neck as you lower your chin. Rest.

Take hold of your chin and this time use your hands to keep it in place. Begin opening your mouth by moving your upper jaw. The whole top of your head will move along with you—the only part that remains still is the chin. Notice what you feel in the back of your neck. Rest.

Slowly begin to move the corners of your lips outward, a little at a time. You can move the corners out a little, and then let them return slowly a few times, each time going a little farther. How far feels comfortable for you? How does the movement of the lips affect the jaw? How do you feel in the moment that your teeth are revealed? How do your eyes feel? Do any thoughts come up? Rest.

Try the same exercise with the corners of the mouth going down. Notice the same things—the jaw, the rest of the face. How is it different for you? Rest.

Notice your tongue. Where is it resting in your mouth? Does one side feel larger than the other? Does your tongue feel like it's in the center or more to one side? Slowly move the tip of your tongue across the back of your upper teeth. Then trace along the back of your lower teeth. Now reverse the motion. After you have circled, press your tongue against your closed teeth a few times. Rest.

Slowly begin to pucker your lips as if you were reach for a kiss or to suck on a straw. Pucker and release several times. How does your jaw respond in this motion? Try actually sucking in, as if you were drawing on a straw. Rest.

Return to your jaw and lower it slightly. Let it move very gently a little to the left, and then to the right. What does your tongue do? Which direction of the jaw is easier? Does it go straight across or does it click around? Rest.

How does your mouth feel now? When you're ready, go to the mirror and take a look at your face. Do you see anything new? Take some time to write down your observations. As you go about your day, notice how many times you remember what your lips are saying besides the actual words you are speaking.

THE TELLTALE BLUSH

I don't deserve any credit for turning the other cheek as my tongue is always in it.

FLANNERY O'CONNOR

It's a simple physiological fact that when you are emotionally aroused—whether angry, embarrassed, or excited, blood rushes to the face in varying degrees, betraying your emotional state. Caressing someone's cheek indicates a level of tenderness or sentimentality. And to slap a cheek is the ultimate offense. Your cheeks tell stories and they respond to what you experience in the world of the emotions. There are, however, ruddy-cheeked people who are struggling with high blood pressure and even levels of toxicity that are forcing the blood to the face (think of the flush of a drunk). Therefore, when reading cheeks it is important to study the whole person.

We read cheeks: "Her cheeks reddened with shame," "The color slowly rose in his cheeks as he listened angrily," and so on. A kiss on the cheek from a loving grandparent suffuses a child with love. Our contemporary "air kisses" pretend at emotion. And a chaste kiss on the cheek from a potential lover is an indication of romantic interest, not yet daring to make that intimate connection with the vital, sexual part of the mouth.

THE SMELL OF THINGS

Fee, fie, foe, fum, I smell the blood of an Englishman!

THE GIANT FROM "JACK AND THE BEANSTALK"

We don't often think of the nose as expressive, and perhaps that's why we often miss the cues that noses offer us. Our nose is a key tool for orientation. We are attracted to the smell of Mom's cooking; we turn away from unpleasant odors. Perhaps you can remember watching Bugs Bunny cartoons where Bugs is literally wafted across the air, dragged by his nose toward an intoxicating smell. And there is a tiny bit of iron in your nose that acts as a little compass, literally helping you orient yourself, if you can really pay attention, toward the North Pole. Although most of us no longer rely on our sense of smell for survival, it has been shown that the sense of smell can evoke emotional responses quickly.

According to David Givens, PhD, director of the Center for Nonverbal Studies at Spokane University, "Like a whiff of smelling salts, a sudden feeling may jolt the mind. The force of a mood is reminiscent of a smell's intensity (e.g., soft and gentle, pungent, or overpowering), and similarly permeates and fades as well. The design of emotion cues, in tandem with the forebrain's olfactory prehistory, suggests that *the sense of smell is the neurological model for our emotions.*" In Buddhism our emotions are categorized as either desire or aversion. There is no organ that responds as quickly to attraction and repulsion as the nose. Givens posits that the animal brain orients toward food, friend, or foe based on olfactory cues, which eventually led to the connection of emotion to smell.

Even infants will turn away or screw up their noses at the smell of rotten eggs. Flaring nostrils, pinched nostrils, or a wrinkled nose are all expressions that reflect an emotional reaction. "Something smells funny about her attitude." "I smell money." "This deal stinks!"

Since we have a tendency to assume that the nose just sits there "as plain as the nose on your face," the expressions of the nose can be difficult to study. Therefore different people will find they are good with different expressions of the nose. It's hard to believe, for example, that a person's habitual use of the nose could result in pinched nostrils, giving a prissy quality to the face. Or that the nose could get slightly wrinkled upward, creating a critical, disgusted look. Many people also have sinus problems and breathing issues because of tension in the nasal passages themselves. This in turn affects the resonance and tone of the voice and can have an impact on other organs of communication (strained throat, tight jaw, and so on).

While it's true that some of the shape of your nose is genetic, what you do with it over a lifetime informs others of your personality. Thus, for example, we speak of a cruel nose or a sensuous nose.

Do You Know Your Nose?

Stand in front of a mirror and notice whether your nostrils are flared, wide, or contracted and pinched. Sometimes it's impossible to know until you explore the movement of your nose. If you are old enough to have some character lines, notice which lines are most prominent across the bridge of your nose, lateral or vertical. Lateral lines indicate nostril flaring or raising—emotions like anger, disgust, and excitement are easy for you. Vertical lines indicate compression—worry, cruelty, discrimination (as in a discriminating nose) are a few emotions associated with contraction.

Now play a little. Try flaring your nostrils. With or without nose wrinkling, this expression indicates levels of excitement or passion. A wolf in a singles' bar might be revealed by his flaring nostrils. Now keep them flared and raise them up. Does your forehead wrinkle? What happens to your eyes? Your mouth? It is very difficult to isolate the muscles of the nose from the rest of the face. This is one reason why we don't often realize that the nose is really the creator of the expression. Even the flaring of just one nostril changes the face. Now try the opposite. Pinch your nostrils together. You may find that one of these directions is easier than the other. People who find it easy to pinch their nostrils may find it easier in life to close off from others. Judgment, contempt, even cruelty can be read in pinched nostrils, depending on how they relate to the rest of the nose and the face. Now close your eyes and just feel your nose. Does it feel more alive to you now?

PINOCCHIO, RUDOLPH, AND MUNCHKINS . . .

Perhaps one reason the story of Pinocchio has had such an enduring effect on us is its basis in fact. According to Alan R. Hirsch, MD, neurological director of the Smell and Taste Treatment Research Foundation, the nose contains erectile tissues that engorge when a person is lying. In psychology this is called the "Pinocchio Effect." We are told that you can tell when a person is lying from mannerisms such as nose or eye rubbing. But unless you know the person, these cues can be misread. What is infinitely more interesting is to begin to listen to your own nose—can you become sensitive enough to respond to its swelling and relaxing, its sensitivities and reactions? Can you sense when you are lying—either to others or yourself?

Rudolph the Red-Nosed Reindeer was embarrassed by his shiny red nose. He was exposed, vulnerable, and rejected by others. If you've ever had the opportunity to put on the clown's red nose, you have experienced the nakedness of the fool. My husband once asked his serious parents to pose for a portrait wearing clown noses. They sat there staring at the camera, his mother smiling, his father stone-faced. It is one of the most poignant portraits I've seen. The nose reddens as a result of stress, passion, or over-indulgence. You don't often hear women say, "Oh, he has such a cute red nose." While it is nearly impossible to control the reddening of the nose, you can at least recognize that something is out of balance when the nose is red.

The tension in your nose's expressions interacts with your sinuses, eyes, and jaw. It affects the quality of your voice: nasal, de-nasal (which sounds like clogged sinuses or a Munchkin), and breathy voices are just a few vocal qualities brought to you by the nose.

Karen is a bright, witty woman who came to me with a severely adenoidal voice. She sounded like she had a perpetually stuffy nose; she said that she had always sounded like this. She was prone to severe sinus infections and had had surgery twice for polyps growing in her nose. She came to see me in desperation after she was told she would need surgery again. As we talked, I noticed that she habitually kept squeezing her nose, pushing her voice out of the back of her throat to create a high-pitched, childlike sound. We began working with exercises to open and relax the nose and the quality of breath. Eventually it emerged that Karen, the only girl in a family of boys, had an attack of tonsillitis as a child, which initially created this voice. This happened during a particularly challenging period in her family, and her voice got her a lot of attention and was considered cute. Unconsciously it became Karen's permanent voice, long after she had had her tonsils out and her adenoidal swelling had gone down. As we worked together with exercises similar to the ones that follow, Karen's nose and voice relaxed and her sinus troubles were greatly reduced.

Opening the Nose ❧

Find a comfortable position—either lying down or sitting. Close your eyes and begin to notice how you breathe through your nose. How long is your inhale? Your exhale? Is there a sound as you breathe? Sometimes the sound comes from congestion, as our breath labors through the clogged nasal passages. Sometimes it is tension. Sometimes it's habit from childhood. Many children suffer from respiratory difficulties, and as they grow out of them bad breathing habits remain, so that in many adults mouth breathing and labored breathing affect both the quality of breath and the voice. See if you can begin to alter the pattern of your breathing so that you make absolutely no sound as you breathe. This may cause you to slow down how much air you take in at a time. It may lengthen your inhale or your exhale. Take your time and let the air come in slowly, slowly, then let it out just as silently and slowly. Do this several times, then let it go and rest.

Now cover one nostril and continue this experiment. After doing this several times, switch to the other nostril. You may find that while one nostril works just fine, the other is clogged. If you go very slowly, you will find that the clogged nostril begins to clear up. Remember to try to go as slowly and silently as you can. Then remove your hand and breathe normally for a few minutes.

Lightly place your hand on a part of your nose. Begin to hum and see if you can hum in such a way that you feel your nose vibrating. You can move your hand to different parts of your nose. Hum for a few minutes, then rest and just notice your breath. You can also try closing off one nostril at a time.

After you rest, sense your breathing. Does your nose feel any different? Try speaking and listen to the sound of your voice.

Observing tension in the nose is extremely challenging, but it can be rewarding, especially in difficult social situations. You can follow your nose in understanding where you are comfortable, who you want to interact with, and what they might be trying to communicate with you.

THE WINDOWS OF THE SOUL

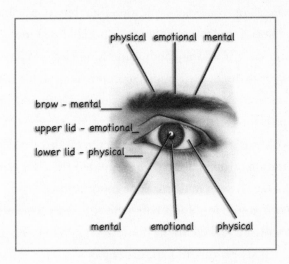

Men judge generally more by the eye than by the hand, for everyone can see and few can feel.
Everyone sees what you appear to be, few really know what you are.

From Niccolò Machiavelli's *The Prince*

I had a professor in college who was a the master of raising one eyebrow—it could look alternately quizzical, condescending, or delighted depending on how the rest of his face joined in. I eventually learned to raise my right eyebrow well, and my left somewhat, but using them in this way has never been an automatic reaction for me. Like the infant with her grandfather's "grief expression," we each have our repertoire of automatic eye expressions: the eyebrows and the eyes express reaction constantly, most of the time without our awareness or intention.

The power of the eyes to communicate is part of our survival strategy. The eyes are light receptors and the movement of the eyes affects our orientation, verticality, and worldview. The pupil enlarges or narrows depending on the amount of light as well as what it is looking at. The basic prime directives, eating and reproduction, are reflected in the movement of the pupil. Sexual arousal enlarges the pupils. In the movie *Kinsey,* Dr. Alfred Kinsey asks a group of students in his first sex studies class, "What organ has the possibility of growing to one hundred times its size?" A flustered young woman sputters, "You have no right to ask me a question like that in mixed company!" Kinsey smiles and says, "My dear, I was talking about the pupil of your eye. You are in for a big disappointment if you were thinking about something else!" Women used to even put belladonna in their eyes to dilate their pupils to make them more attractive. The pupils also enlarge when someone is frightened. So wide eyes with enlarged pupils range in meaning from receptivity to terror.

At one of my workshops I made use of character masks. I did not speak about or explain my interpretation of the masks before I invited the class to explore them. One of the masks was of a face frozen in terror. The mouth is wide open, the eyes wide. An attractive woman with abundant blond hair who dressed provocatively and used her attractiveness to manipulate picked up the mask of fear. When she put the mask on, instead of taking on the body posture of fear, she began tossing her hair and placing herself into coy "come hither" postures, sidling up to men and jutting out her hips. Suddenly the mask of fear had become a sexy bimbo. This woman had interpreted the wide eyes as the wide eyes of an empty-headed sex kitten, the open mouth as an invitation. It showed us all the relationship between sexual conquest and predator/prey. Conversely, small pupils and narrow eyes indicate hostility and distaste. They also create a kind of focus, like taking aim, closing out peripheral vision and therefore distractions—concentration, intensity, and singlemindedness on the goal in front make them seem predatory.

In the Mahabharata, an Indian epic tale about seven divine brothers, the brothers were learning archery from their teacher, Drona. Drona pointed to a bird on a high branch and asked each brother to take aim in turn. "What do you see?" he asked Bhishma.

"I see the bird, the branch he is sitting on, the sky . . ."

Drona pushed Bhishma away. Yudhisithira then took aim. "What do you see?"

"I see the blue feathers on his wing, the scaly bark on the tree." Drona pushed him aside, too, not allowing him to shoot. So it went, from brother to brother, until finally it was Arjuna's turn. Arjuna took aim. "What do you see?" asked Drona.

Arjuna barely moved and muttered, "His eye."

Drona asked again, "What do you see?"

"His eye."

"What else?"

"Nothing, I see nothing but his eye."

"Then shoot!" cried Drona in delight. Arjuna eventually becomes the warrior in the group.

The enlargement and narrowing of the pupil are functions of the autonomic nervous system and therefore are not necessarily in our voluntary control. However, the various expressions that are triggered by the pupil's response can be studied and understood.

Both a wide-eyed stare of terror and the squinting of concentration create limitations. They also affect others, making us uncomfortable. For example, a person with a permanent deer in headlights expression can seem tense, frightened, or even belligerent (if they are hiding their fear). On the other hand, when you meet someone with soft, relaxed eyes, you feel reassured that this person can take care of the situation. When the eyes are relaxed, one is actually able to see more—a bigger picture. Our reptile brain feels reassured because it is able to scan. The eyes can then gaze upon any situation—nothing interferes with looking and turning the head or taking an action. The movement of the eyes often commands the response of the head in turning, mobilizing the entire body. Someone with bulging eyes often has tension in the neck, which makes a quick escape and an ability to "see everything" more difficult. She has to figure out clever ways of negotiating through challenging situations because the eyes can't help. Someone who has narrowed his eyes can only go forward toward his object of desire—everything else is in his way.

Isaac originally came to see me because of headaches and back pain. Isaac's most outstanding feature was his eyes. They were beautiful, dark gypsy eyes, but they looked like they were about to jump out of his head. As he spoke, sometimes his eyes would get even wider as he described a work situation or an event. It occurred to me that some of Isaac's headaches might be the result of his huge eyes. We worked through movement, not just of the eyes, but how the eyes connect to other movements of the body. He confided that he had trouble with relationships, that men either took advantage of his generosity or used him until they found someone they really loved, then dumped him. His eyes seemed to convey someone needy and easy. It also happened that he is the youngest in his family, Mommy's little boy. His wide-eyed expression perhaps could have originated as a look of wonder. Or it may have been an unconscious choice to keep the doe eyes of a child's face. In any case, once Isaac was able to relax his eyes his freedom of movement increased. He became more discriminating about the men he chose. His eyes still widen when he talks about his mom, however.

Your eyes play a major part in keeping you balanced as you move through space. The eye muscles connect to neurons that determine distance, dimension, and orientation. This neural network joins with your vestibular system (which keeps you vertical). When you faint or go to sleep, where do your eyes go? If you guessed that they roll up into the head, you're right. What is the relation of this movement to loss of verticality?

The eyes do more than just see, and you don't see with just your eyes. Scientist Paul Bach-y-Rita has done some amazing experiments with how the rest of the body sees. By attaching electrodes to the tongue, for example, a blindfolded person in a special room that muffles all sound can still easily catch a ball rolling across a table.

Your eye expressions are connected to the rest of your face; it is very difficult to isolate an eye expression and know exactly what it is saying. But there are some simple ways to explore your repertoire of eye expressions. Your eyes, like your hands, have a direct link to many brain functions. Delsarte placed the eyes in the mental zone. Your eyes reveal your thoughts; hence Pliny's expression that the eyes are the "windows of the soul."

Delsarte also saw the eyes as a microcosm of the entire body, so he divided each part of the eye into his mental, emotional, and physical trinities, as illustrated at the beginning of this section.

The Eyes' Repertoire

Actor Michael Caine practiced not blinking because he believes that blinking in a close-up diminishes the power of the shot. The Italian film actor Giancarlo Giannini once said that he spent an hour a day in front of his mirror doing eye exercises in order to communicate his emotions more effectively and with clarity of intention. The expressions of the eyes are rarely interpreted out of context, but much still can be learned from studying the eyes, their movement and their habits.

You can try the following exercise with or without a mirror. These are just a few of the isolations used by actors while training to use their eyes.

1. Widen your eyes and then relax them several times.
2. With your eyes wide, look left, then quickly return to a center focal point. Repeat to the right, then up and down.
3. Think of a clock in front of each eye and circle your eye around the numbers. Do it slowly, then quickly, both clockwise and counterclockwise. Then from your center point, shoot your eyes to each hour, returning to the center point. Imagine you're drawing a star with your eyes.
4. Raise and lower your eyebrows several times. As you noticed in the illustration at the beginning of this section, the eyebrow can also be looked at in parts. Then raise the inner brows and lower them. Try to raise and lower the outer brows. Can you raise one brow at a time? Delsarte called the eyebrow "nothing less than the door of intelligence." Suddenly *Star Trek*'s Dr. Spock raising his outer eyebrow takes on a whole new meaning.

Once you have done the movements strictly as an exercise, play with the various positions you have discovered and notice if any evoke familiar or unfamiliar feelings. For example, if your eyes travel diagonally upward, do you feel like you are thinking or imagining? What happens if you add a tilt of the head? In the chapter on the head, I discussed the intimate relationship between the head and eyes. Take some time now to explore the movements of the head in relation to the eyes. You will see that your eyes play a part in any position you put your head into. And each position that your eyes choose expresses an emotion. For example, try lowering your head and rolling your eyes upward. It gives an expression of incredible boredom, and you will soon feel tired.

After playing each time, take some time to note down your experiences. Were there certain expressions that came easily to you? Others that you recognize from friends or family? What did it feel like to try on an unfamiliar look?

After a few days, take your observations out into the field. Notice if you can sense what your eyes are doing when you engage in conversations with others. Can you read other people's eyes?

Oh, Really?

This exercise is much more fun if you do it with a friend. Using your eyes, eyelids, and eyebrows, see how many different ways you can say "Oh really" to each other. Feel free to allow your voice and body to participate in the gesture, but let the eyes lead the expression. Thus narrowed eyes and a furrowed brow would create a much different meaning than if the head is turned away and the eyes are glancing sideways!

Relaxing the Eyes ›

Your eyes are held in place by three sets of muscles that let your eyes track whatever objects come into your line of vision. By learning to relax these muscles, you can soften your gaze and, consequently, improve your vision. Relaxing the eyes also often helps relieve headaches and neck tension, since the eye muscles are so connected to head and neck movements.

You can do this exercise either lying down or sitting.

Close your eyes. Cup your right hand over your right eye, your fingers on your forehead pointing slightly to the left. Place your left hand over your left eye. Do not press on the eyeballs. Keeping your breath soft, notice what is going on in front of your eyes. Is it completely black? Are there patchy areas of light? Maybe even some little bursts of light? This is your excited visual cortex trying to make sense of the information. Look into the blackness and see if you can find the darkest patch of black. Try to imagine that blackness spreading across your entire field of vision. Keeping your eyes closed, let go and rest.

Now imagine a Ping-Pong ball sitting on the bridge of your nose. Let it float away in front of your face. Keep looking at it in your mind's eye as it floats into the distance, getting smaller, until it's just a little white dot. Then gradually let it come back. Let it land on the bridge of your nose. Repeat this movement slowly about five times. Then, still in your mind's eye, throw that Ping-Pong ball away, far into deep space. Let it return just as quickly. Repeat that several times, then rest.

Slowly open your eyes. How does the world look now?

TOWARD A NEW YOU

Paul Ekman found that his mood was profoundly affected by spending time with a certain expression on his face. Choose a few moments during your day—while on the phone, at work, or with your children—and notice the expression on your face. Slowly, intentionally, let a smile spread. See if you can stay smiling for at least one minute. Notice what happens to your state as well as to your relationship to the situation you are in.

You will discover, as you go deeper into the study of your face, that there are many muscular connections between your expressions and the postures of your body. Like the link between the pelvis and the jaw, the face will be reflected throughout yourself. Because we are such a face-oriented culture, I've included a lot of material in this chapter. Allow yourself plenty of time to investigate the nuances and connections—it will be worth the effort.

Exploration Checklist

☐ Take some time in front of a mirror and examine where your lines are. How do they correlate with the mask you present to the world?

☐ Try the "I Forgot" exercise, either alone or with a friend.

☐ Explore the nine basic expressions of the mouth.

☐ Investigate the movement of your mouth and jaw in the somatic exercise "Lip (and Jaw) Service."

☐ Examine your nose's possibilities of expression.

☐ Learn how your nose, breath, and sinuses are connected in the exercise "Opening the Nose."

☐ Try the actors' eye isolations and write about your experience. Then try to observe your eye movements in life.

☐ Do the "Oh, Really?" exercise, with a friend if possible.

☐ Do the "Relaxing the Eyes" somatic exploration.

☐ Put on a happy face in "Toward a New You."

Part Three

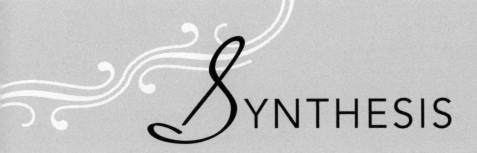

SYNTHESIS

In this section we will begin to integrate the lessons from previous chapters with the aim of an experience of embodiment, to truly inhabit the body. By developing this heightened kinesthetic sense, you will begin to experience combinations of the four components of action: sensing, feeling, thinking, and moving. You will then be able to sense while thinking, feel while moving. In this way you will be more able to clarify and then live your intention.

Ten

PRACTICAL SHAPE-SHIFTING

WHO SHALL I BE TODAY?

We've all had days when, upon looking in the mirror, we seem different. Sometimes it's the shock of seeing wrinkles. Sometimes we are pleased to notice that we look pretty damn good. Sometimes I forget that I am short and feel gigantic, striding down the city streets and sometimes I am a fragile, petite waif. I change along with my self-image, constantly morphing, influenced by outer circumstances, inner attitudes, and others' observations. The human body, while often referred to as a bag of water, is actually mostly oxygen (65 percent). The minerals we each contain, if compacted together, would be about the size of a brick. Our perception of solidity is just that—a perception. Within my skin reside many selves, and each of these selves has a unique body language and ways of approaching the world. My attitudes and attention are all that make the world (and myself) seem solid and unchangeable.

Doing the exercises in this book may have altered your posture, your impression of how you stand and walk, or your experience of your cardinal lines. Each time you have shape-shifted a little bit. There are stories in every culture about shape shifters—from the god Morpheus in Greek mythology to countless fairy tales and Native American legends. While it is intriguing to contemplate the possibility of transforming into an eagle, or even to be able to shift from being a stocky brunette to a willowy blonde, we will emphasize the practical applications in our ordinary lives. A friend put it to me best: "What good will it do my career if I know how to turn into a lion but still can't win the contract?" "Why would I want to be an eagle, when what I really want is a good relationship with a man I love!" "How can I be soft and receptive, strong and assertive, dazzling when necessary?"

THE BIG (AND LITTLE) PICTURE

You can't just change your posture by imposing a new pattern on your old pattern. Each part of your carriage, attitudes, and reactions is the result of years of hard wiring, what we call habits. The saying, "Change one thing and you change everything" can be both positive and negative. Without understanding your habit and the impact it has on your system, you could be creating more damage than good. Feldenkrais maintained that if you try to eradicate or alter a habit or aspect of the posture you often end up with a worse habit in its place. This is because each aspect of your behavior is part of an over-all pattern that is you. By trying to eliminate one thing you don't like, you create con-flict in the overall pattern. For example, if you don't understand why you have the habit of smoking, and then force yourself to stop, you may substitute smoking with overeat-ing or you may become extremely cranky.

The previous chapters contained many examples of how patterns manifest in every aspect of behavior. Feldenkrais stressed that one should never look at parts. During a lecture he once said, "I say I love *you,* I don't say I love your eyelid, or the right side of your rump, or your pinkie. I love *you.*" When a person looks at you, they don't just notice your eyebrows, or the way your right leg turns out slightly. They look at the whole self, even if all the details are not absorbed consciously. Yet these details are what create the whole. In order to effectively read others, as well as to be able to understand your own pattern, you need to be able to experience both. This is how you can begin to clarify mixed signals—details in your posture that belie your intentions.

Peter Brook, one the world's foremost theater directors, spoke in one of his lectures about the importance of clarity of intention by employing the metaphor of a tightrope walker. If I am only fixed on my goal, I may miss the wire and fall. Or I may not see the runaway trapeze swing heading my way in time to protect myself. If, however, I am so intent on noticing the audience or the act in the other ring, I can also lose my balance. When I become so concentrated on putting one foot in front of another, I again lose sight of my goal and miss an aspect of the big picture that is necessary for my success. It is important to have an inclusive attention that allows you to perceive the big picture and details simultaneously.

If your goal is to be a sexier you, or to become more assertive at your job, or to shift the anger you feel toward your spouse, this becomes the other end of your tight rope. It is the big picture and forms the background for all of your manifestations. As you journey toward your goal, you can begin to see more and more details about yourself that can help or hinder your progress. By learning to hold an awareness of your goal alongside clarity of the details of your body language, you can begin to choose the path that will lead you in the direction of your aim. But until you can see both the details and the big aim at the same time, you will get lost in either one or the other. This inability to see the forest for the trees is one reason many people start out with one intention and find themselves years later living in the opposite of the dream they held for themselves.

"Every Move You Make" ⟩

Whenever I hear that classic song by the Police, I think of myself. "I'll be watching you." What is it like to watch myself? To be able to feel my integrity, understand my walk, see the details and the big picture of what I call "me"? Is it possible for my actions to be congruent with my intentions?

Create a space large enough for you to be able to lie down with your arms and legs outstretched, like an X. You should have enough room for your arms to reach both over your head and out to either side. You may want to have a pillow or cushion available to support your head. If lying on the floor is not an option for you, you can do a variation of this lesson by sitting in a chair and doing minimal movements with the legs. Or you can do this exercise lying in bed. Place your arms at your side. While lying on your back, take a moment to sense your shape. As in other scans we have done, notice what is comfortable, what presses into the floor. But also notice what your right side feels like in comparison to your left. Perhaps one side feels larger or more alive. Or maybe the impression is about how the two sides contact the floor differently. Can you sense the shape of your face?

Lie on your left side. Bend your knees as if you were sitting in a chair. Bend your arms so that they look like a mirror of the legs.

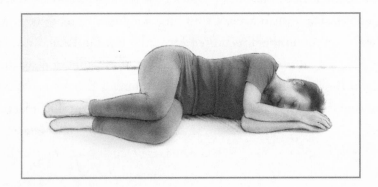

Place your right hand on your forehead. Now slowly fold your head, right arm, and right elbow down toward your right knee. At the same time, bring your right knee up toward your right elbow. This should be a small movement; it's not about touching. Let your leg slide, not lift, so that you are not straining your back to move the leg. Gently fold, then unfold back to your neutral space several times.

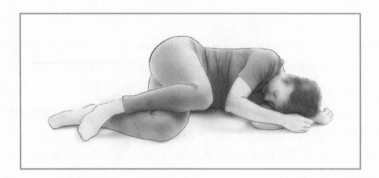

The action is folding and unfolding. But how do you do this? For a moment, turn your attention to your elbow and knee—just those two parts. What are they doing? Are they creating the folding? How do they participate? What is the relationship between the shoulder and the hip? As you do the movement, imagine that you are looking at yourself from above with a special lens. Allow this lens to zoom in to just observing the shoulder and hip, then zoom out and take in the entire action. Play with this lens for a few minutes, alternately looking at the details and then the big picture.

Roll onto your back and rest.

As you are resting, return to sensing your shape. Is there something different on each side? Can you identify the sensation? Roll back onto your left side.

This time, begin to *unfold*. Stretch your right leg away from your head, look upward, and reach your right arm above your head.

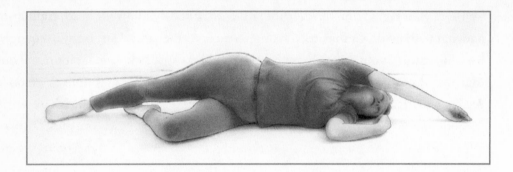

Can you sense what your hand and foot are doing to make this action occur? Shine your lens on the detail of your breathing. What does your torso do as you breathe? Are you able to include this detail in your big picture? In other words, can you sense your torso and the action of unfolding simultaneously? After completing the movement a few times, roll onto your back and rest.

By the way, how did you roll onto your back? Where did your attention go?

Roll back onto your left side. This time try both motions—the folding and the unfolding.

Once again rest on your back. As you're resting, notice your mind. Are there thoughts or is the mind quiet? Are the thoughts connected to your sensations? Emotions? Or are you thinking about dinner? Just as there is a foreground and a background to your physical picture, there is a foreground and background to your mental and emotional states. By paying attention you can begin to notice thoughts or feelings in the background of your mind that are participating in your actions. Like the elbow and the knee, we don't always notice how these thoughts are participating in the big picture of how we do things. These are the background emotions that we have been exploring in earlier chapters.

Continue to lie on your back and imagine rolling onto your *right side* and doing the same movement of folding and unfolding with your left arm and leg. As you picture this, can you "see" the details involved in rolling to the side? How do you do it? What will the parts do to enact folding and unfolding? Once you see the movement clearly, execute it. Was it the way you imagined it would be? Was there tension somewhere? An unnoticed part? An overlooked detail? Was the overall quality what you expected? Play with reimagining and then actually trying the sequence both of folding/unfolding and rolling to your back and back to your side. Can you find a way to do this without tension or straining?

This process of observing the larger picture on a physical scale and where small tensions interfere is the same process that can help you to clarify how you present yourself to the world. As you lie on your back and rest at the end of your exploration, take note of how your shape has begun to shift as the result of attending to your quality of ease and movement. Then take a few minutes standing and walking to see if there is something clearer in your perception of your shape as it moves through space.

Expanding Your Vision

Now that you have looked at the whole picture of yourself in the laboratory of your room, you can take the experiment into the world. Here are several ways to try:

1. Observe someone—at a restaurant, in a waiting room, shopping. Take note of how they use their parts. If you have a notebook, all the better. What are the arms doing? The head? Where is the pelvis? Then note down your impression of this person's character/mood. What is it about that person's parts that contribute to this overall impression? What stands out? If you can hear them talking, what is congruent or incongruent in their words versus their actions?

2. Now observe the same thing in yourself. Take your imaginary lens with you to a social situation. It can be as simple as the checkout counter at a grocery store or as challenging as a party. Take mental snapshots of your details. How do you stand? Where are your hands? Shoulders? Are you breathing? Note the details and the big pictures. If you were someone else looking at you, what would the impression be? Try this several times, writing down your

impressions as soon as possible. As you continue to do this experiment, you will see, like the old Polaroids, a picture emerging that tells your story.

3. How do you translate these observations into tools for achieving your goals? Go back to your goal worksheets from the beginning of the book. Even if you haven't looked at them since you first filled them out, pull them out now. If you never even started, that's okay too—you can begin now. If you have been working with the worksheets, sort your pages into long-term or short-term goals. Which ones do you feel you have accomplished in the course of working through this book? Congratulations! Put them aside for now and look at the ones that still seem out of reach. Write these goals down again on separate pieces of paper. If you didn't do the first worksheet, just begin with this. Then you may be motivated to go back and investigate differently.

Give each goal a full page. If you have been working with the worksheets, you may find that you have some new goals as well. They can be long-range goals ("I want to write a book," "I want to move to Europe") or short-term ones ("I want to be a good conversationalist at the party tonight," "I want to have a civil discussion with my misbehaving son when he gets home"). Then write down some strategies that you can begin to explore in order to get there. These can be physical ("I will be aware of my breath as I call the writing coach," "I will sense my jaw as I speak to my son"). They can be practical ("I will look for employment agencies in Italy that specialize in my line of work," "I will introduce myself to three new people at the party").

As you move toward your goal, use these pages to note down the ways in which you interfere with and the ways in which you clarify your intentions. Whether it is a short-term or a long-term goal, you may find parallels in how you approach things. By re-examining your goals in this fashion, you may have new insights into hidden motives. And you may discover that these interferences are connected to the kind of efforts you have been making.

RELAX!

I'm so tense, now when I'm calm I get nervous!

FROM A POSTCARD FOUND IN
A MEMPHIS DRUGSTORE

As you become better at observing the details that make up your big picture, you will become aware of how much of your body language is the result of tension. It is so much easier to rationalize, justify, and soothe the ego with explanations than to look honestly and say, "This is what I do." The paradox is that there is a liberating effect when you finally admit this to yourself. You will see how much unnecessary tension has gone into maintaining your personal patterns of self-deception and self-sabotage. Tension is a dead giveaway that some part of your behavior is not congruent with your intentions. It can manifest itself in a small, perhaps even invisible, fashion—a habitual curling of the toes, for example. Or it can travel around the whole self—held breath, tense shoulders, frozen pelvis, a pained smile. Others sense this tension and they respond in kind.

Unnecessary tension is not inevitable. It is not our natural state, but a habit that interferes with effective function and our true intention. In terms of our study of body language, this tension is part of your pattern of communication.

It's not that our muscles shouldn't work. After all, if we didn't have muscles we'd just be a pile of bones on the floor. Your muscles are working constantly to keep you vertical, the dance with gravity that only ends when you flop down on the couch or yield to your bed (although even then many people continue to grip their buttocks, hunch their shoulders, and grit their teeth!). And sometimes illness and injury create patterns of tension in the body—trying to support or protect you in ways that are difficult to overcome. The tonus in an arm that has been affected by a stroke, for example, may never go away, but there are ways to work with it to reduce the discomfort. The tension in the shoulders and around the neck after a whiplash accident is perfectly normal. However, when your body turns it into a habit, it can affect your outlook on life. At that point the constant tensing of your neck has become part of your body language.

While we all want to be relaxed, confident, and flexible, the truth is that life is constantly creating situations that invite tension. In my book *What Are You Afraid Of? A Body/Mind Guide to Courageous Living,* I speak at length about the relationship of tension to fear in our daily lives. But tension can also indicate inner conflict, determination, and enthusiasm. Whenever you notice that you are not centered along your plumb line, you can be sure that tension is playing a part in your carriage and your communication. The question becomes "Is that tension serving you, or are you serving it?"

Victor is a very careful, methodical man who works in an accounting firm and is known for his efficiency and competence. His life is rigidly programmed—what time he eats, the exact amount of food and coffee he allows himself. He allots himself two beers a week— no more, no less. He hates to deviate from any aspect of his schedule—for example, he walks to work even in the most inclement weather, because that is his "time to walk."

Victor, however, has another side—a passionate devotion to playing the guitar. He began to play while he was a teenager during the heyday of Jimi Hendrix and the electric guitar revolution. Every Tuesday, Thursday, and Saturday, at his precisely scheduled times, Victor sits down to play. Lately he has felt the stagnation of repeating the songs from his youth, so he started taking guitar lessons to increase the range of his repertoire. This has meant practice and learning new fingering techniques. In addition, his teacher has encouraged him to play in public, to join a band in order to feel the power of ensemble music.

Victor came to me because of incredible stiffness in his neck and lower back. As we worked together, some of the stiffness disappeared, but he still felt pain after playing. I went to see him perform at a local open mike concert with the group he had joined. He sat hunched over his guitar, his eyes straining at the singer, his head protruding forward. When something was up to him—a change in rhythm, a guitar solo, a flourish, his shoulders rose to his ears, his eyes squinted as if he was trying to see something, and his elbow went flying out away from the guitar. All of his efforts made the music more difficult, not

easier, to play. In addition, the audience perhaps was not as able to enjoy the music com-
pletely because his tension made us uneasy.

Victor's pattern connected to an extremely old habit formed in childhood that had be-
come invisible to him. By beginning to study his habits, he slowly was able to become
more comfortable while playing. He began to notice parts of this same pattern in other as-
pects of his life. By experimenting with his physical tension he has also become less rigid in
his schedule.

Whether your tension is the result of old trauma or injury or an ongoing psychological habit, you can begin to work with it by developing your awareness. In the beginning of the book you did a postural scan to discover your personal neutral. While
working on the exercises in the book you may have discovered new ways of carrying/
using yourself that felt easier. I also addressed how certain expressions communicate
different attitudes toward others. As you become more aware of your postural habits,
you will also start to recognize which of these are habitual tensions. The following is a
checklist of some of the more common ways habitual tension influences your body language. Often these tension habits work in concert—clenched jaw and clenched buttocks, for example. Notice how many times a day you catch yourself in one of these
manifestations.

Forehead: Wrinkled, furrows in the brow
Eyes: Squinting or very wide
Mouth: Lips tight, jaw clenched, tongue biting
Neck: Head projecting forward
Shoulders: Hunched, rounded, unmoving
Hands: Fingers clenched, stretched; picking at cuticles, biting nails,
    wringing hands
Chest: Shallow breath, stiff ribs
Spine: Stiffness, soreness

Buttocks: Clenched

Legs: Knees locked; gripping calves and/or ankles

Feet: Curling toes up or down

Remember that each time you tense and each time you relax in your interaction with others, you are communicating with them. By practicing awareness of your habits, you will begin to change how you feel, and consequently how others will feel about you.

Several years ago I was an artist-in-residence in the South Bronx. It was a voluntary after-school program for at-risk eighth graders. It was the kind of school where hats were not allowed so you couldn't conceal a weapon underneath. The undercurrent of chaos and violence was underscored by the presence of armed security guards in the hallways. The students were a simmering, brooding lot just waiting for an excuse to explode.

I usually showed up for class with enough ideas for four hours of material because I never knew which ones would catch their fancy and which ones would utterly bomb. Finding activities that would engage the students was an ongoing challenge. One day tension filled the room as I walked in. The students were distracted by issues from the school day and all my brilliant suggestions were rebuffed. The class quickly spun out of control—a couple of boys began running around, some of the girls tried to leave the classroom, and crumpled pieces of paper flew through the air. "Quiet!" I tried shouting, to no avail. The minute I'd get one boy into his seat, a fight would erupt on the other side of the room. I was in a maelstrom of chaos. I felt hysteria mounting in me, a desire to stamp my feet and shout, to threaten them with discipline. Suddenly I saw my own body language. My fists were clenched, my shoulders were by my ears. My lower back was in spasm and my eyebrows were deeply furrowed. I stopped and took a breath. And just stood there. I relaxed my hands, softened my knees. I gave up the pretense of being in charge of the class. As I stood there, softly breathing, the class slowly quieted. One by one they stopped their acting out and sat down. Within minutes they all were quietly looking at me. At that moment our true working relationship began.

ATTITUDE ADJUSTMENT

There are many exercises in this book that explore your relationship to your carriage, your walk, your gestures. Take some time to go back and explore some of the exercises again, this time looking at them from the perspective of your tensions. Take note of your habitual postures and expressions and notice for yourself how much tension is required to maintain these positions.

Try to experiment with seeing your tensions in your interactions with other people. See what happens in an argument, for example, or if you can sense your tensions as you talk. Intentionally changing one aspect of an attitude—opening a clenched fist or taking a deep breath, for example—can shift the entire posture and change the entire interaction.

TOWARD A NEW YOU

Go back through the previous chapters and look at the "Toward a New You" exercises at the end of each chapter. Did you do them or just read them and nod? If you did them, what was your response to reading them again? If you did the exercises again today, would you feel something different? Are you willing to try them again without an expectation of the results? Start with your favorites. Notice the ones you want to avoid. Then relate these experiences to some of the ideas suggested earlier in this chapter.

Exploration Checklist

☐ Do the "Every Move You Make" movement exploration and notice the foreground and background of your shape as you move and as you lie still.

☐ Expand your vision: Take your observations into your life, noticing the big and little pictures in other people's postures as well as your own as you interact with others.

☐ Take the time to review your worksheets and/or write down and work with some of your own goals and how you can move toward them.

☐ Study your characteristic tensions.

☐ Go back through the book and find a movement exploration that relates to the tension in the part of the body you noticed.

☐ Experiment with changing one aspect of a tension habit in your life, in a conversation or while working, for example.

Eleven

EMBODYING COMPASSION

Fair and softly goes far.

Miguel de Cervantes

You are in a meeting that is not going well. The sweat is forming under your collar and your irritation level is rising. Your boss is clutching his pen and there is a slight twitch starting in his left eye. He's not happy either. You might raise your shoulders, clench your teeth, and continue to demand your way. He will curl his toes, narrow his eyes, and eventually say no. The Dalai Lama has said, "When you are angry at your enemy, you make him happy, because he sees that you are suffering." How can understanding body language help in your relationships? What is the process of studying your own reactions to another's body language in order to get what you want—either from the person or from the relationship itself? When you recognize that your body language is part of the equation, you can change both your state *and* the state of the person you are facing, with a positive result. Many spiritual disciplines speak about this elusive skill of embodying compassion, but few offer concrete, physical steps for working with the idea beyond meditative practice. While mindfulness and meditation are extremely useful approaches to learning compassion and developing attention to self and others, it is useful to have a few somatic strategies as well.

This chapter aims to begin a bigger investigation. What is our true potential? What occurs when an individual intentionally chooses to adopt the body language of love and tenderness rather than defensiveness and fear? Is such a choice even possible in certain circumstances? Instead of being at the mercy of reactivity, it is possible to monitor your emotional reactions by using your body language as a reference point? Paul Ekman called this process reflective appraisal—a way of interrupting the automatic functioning of the emotions. Buddhists call it mindfulness. G. I. Gurdjieff called it self-observation.

Feldenkrais observed that the body is the easiest, most concrete object you can access with your attention. For example, you and your spouse are in the beginning of an argument, but you don't realize you are getting angry. Your spouse says, "Why are you angry?"

At which point you huff and puff and say, "Angry? I'm not angry!"

"Then why are you raising your voice?"

Your mate may well have asked why are your eyes narrowed, or your lips tight, or your shoulders raised? But often these cues are too subtle for others to notice, especially in an emotional moment. You know now how different parts of the body participate in the manifestation of emotion. You have begun to notice them in yourself—they are concrete. Unlike emotions that can be denied and thoughts that can be confused, physical attitude is objective. You can't say your lips are relaxed when they are tight. You can't say your breath is easy when it is shallow. Beginning to observe your physical state in an encounter is the first step toward being able to choose a stance or demeanor that can change your interaction from a confrontation to a win-win.

Most of the exercises in this chapter require a partner. Sometimes this partner will be unaware that you are experimenting; in fact, sometimes this is better. Other exercises are best done when both people are committed to working together, open and willing to listen to each other's feedback. By working with a friend, you can practice the powers of observation necessary to recognize the subtle cues that affect the balance between compassion and resentment.

I AM THOU

We unconsciously respond to other people's body language because we all own the same repertoire of movements. We clash or resonate with those whose postures are either a reflection of or a response to our own. We recognize lovers in a restaurant because of the way they unconsciously reflect each other's actions: She leans forward, he leans forward, he sips his wine, she picks up her glass, they laugh almost simultaneously. When experiencing antipathy toward another person, it is often because our adversary is unconsciously reflecting some similar quality of our own that we have suppressed. It's extremely difficult to recognize and acknowledge that I might harbor just the very qualities that irritate me about another person!

One of the participants at a weeklong professional workshop I attended was Ted, a bombastic, macho businessman who had a brilliant mind and a completely obnoxious personality. Besides his penchant for pontificating, he had the habit of constantly clucking, as if he were clearing postnasal drip from his throat. Ted sat in a slouchy manner, often with his arm draped familiarly around the back of another person's chair, as if he owned the chair and its occupant. Periodically he would fart loudly. Even more maddening was that women would flock to him. They didn't seem to care at all about his bodily function habits. But I would grit my teeth and avoid his eyes whenever he tried to address me. I asked myself what it was about this guy that was setting me on edge. Why should I care that he seemed to be a love object to others in spite of his grotesque behavior? And why did I flush when he flattered me?

I tried to study myself in the face of these contradictions. To my chagrin and surprise I realized that I resented his manifestations because I was jealous. How many times had I suppressed the desire to belch or fart because I was in polite society? Yet here was someone who not only did it with impunity, but no one seemed to resent him for it! In fact, people found him attractive. His coarseness was only one aspect of his obviously sensual personality that attracted people of both sexes to be around him. Once I was able to accept myself in the presence of Ted, I was able to enjoy both him and myself at the event.

Reflections

When does mirroring a person help an interaction? When does it escalate problems? Can mirroring someone intentionally change the dynamic of the conversation? How is that different from *unconscious* reflection? This exercise usually requires spontaneity—while you can discuss it in advance with a friend or mate, it creates an artificiality in the interaction. You will still get a lot out of it, though, and it is often difficult to try it out outside of an artificial arrangement. One solution is to create an intention if you know you are about to address a difficult situation.

The famous hypnotherapist Milton Erickson was once asked to help with a difficult patient at a mental institution. It seemed this patient spoke only gibberish, and although the staff suspected he understood them, there never seemed to be any communication. This patient had a pattern of sitting on a particular bench every day at noon. Erickson began to appear at the bench at the same time. Every day the patient would jabber to him in his gibberish language. Erickson answered in kind—jabbering away nonsensically. After about a week, the patient turned to Erickson with an exasperated air and said, "What is wrong with you? Can't you speak English?"

Before leaving the house, or before entering a building, make an intention to try one of the following exercises with another person. Each one will have a different effect. Try it in different interactions—with a grocery store clerk, with a friend, with someone you have problems with.

1. Notice how the other person is sitting or standing and carefully adjust yourself to a mirror image of that same posture. Notice if the person shifts, gets more or less comfortable, or changes the nature of what he or she is saying. Notice how you feel in his posture.

2. Notice how a person is using her hands. Carefully, subtly, include some of her gestures in your responses.

BLENDING

In the martial art aikido the term *irimi tenkan* literally translated means "enter and turn." It is a way of blending with the adversary. As he attacks, you enter into the attack and then turn so that you are both facing the same direction—as if you too wish to see the other's point of view. Sometimes the two partners actually seem to be taking the same position—hands flying up into the air, entering into each other's space. But suddenly they have traded places, and in the next moment one of them has been "redirected," which in the case of aikido means he has landed on the floor. To practice this in relationships, you sometimes must be willing to change your body language so that you can enter into the other's atmosphere and see what they are saying. Sometimes it seems like a reflection because you are meeting that person on the same ground, you are using that mirroring posture to turn things around. Sometimes it means that you have to take an apparently opposite tack, a complementary posture in order for them to feel comfortable.

Betty, a student in one of my classes, shared that sometimes she wasn't aware when she was depressed or anxious. She'd be walking down the street or seated in an office when suddenly someone, usually male, would cheerily and heartily say to her, "Hey! Cheer up! Smile!" Or even more irritating, "Relax!" She remarked that usually this made her angry and defensive instead of achieving the desired effect.

While our intentions may be the best when we act jovial with someone, especially someone we care about who seems like they're in a funk, this will rarely cheer her up. Here is where you can "enter and turn" by apparently mirroring behavior. Notice if the chest is collapsed, what the sound of the voice is, and if you can, pay attention to that person's breath. Allow yourself to receive by also softening your chest. Remember that a soft chest is not always a sign of weakness; it is also one of receptivity. As you open yourself to receive from that person, you are inviting her to share with you. Let your voice be soft as well. As you listen to her, also listen to your breath. As you continue to breathe fully and quietly, the rhythm of your breath will affect her mood. As her breath improves, you both will be able to sit straighter, allowing the solar plexus to function more freely. Take the time to agree with her and you will be surprised at the result. You will have changed her posture and her mood by entering into her space and then turning her energy around.

Mirroring anger rarely helps defuse the other person's anger. Court jesters often used this tack, exaggerating (following the yes!) all the manifestations of anger at some silly thing so that others could recognize and laugh at themselves. Of course on occasion it would backfire and the court jester ended up in the dungeon or worse. Certainly humor is a useful tool in the face of anger, but it is often difficult to shift in the right way—so that the angry person doesn't feel like the object of ridicule. It's like the person telling Betty to relax. Often if you tell someone, "Hey, don't be angry," the answer will be either "I AM NOT ANGRY!" or "Who you calling angry?" Instead of defusing the situation, you have escalated it. Marshall Rosenberg, the author of *Non-Violent Communication*, calls this "talking from fear." You then feel threatened by his aggressive behavior, so you respond more aggressively. You go back and forth, and soon you have escalated into a fight, when all he wanted was a little understanding.

Terry Dobson was one of the first Americans to study aikido in Japan, and he was instrumental in spreading its popularity in the United States. He wrote a short story about an encounter in a Japanese subway in which an angry drunk entered the car and Dobson, eager to try out his newly acquired martial arts skills, confronted him. The tension mounted and Dobson was ready to deck the drunk. At that point a little old man spoke to the drunk, invited him to sit down beside him, and began commiserating with him about life. Soon the drunk was weeping in the old man's lap. Dobson, ashamed, realized that he had seen aikido—also called the art of peace—in action.

Like an aikido practitioner, you can find a way to blend with others by receiving what they offer and redirecting it. When someone is aggressive, for example, you may notice that his chest is tense, his breathing is labored. Many times it's difficult to find the right words to say. And even if you know you should be understanding, your heart is beating and your own fight or flight reactions have been triggered. These are the times to return to the body. Instead of reflecting aggression back at him, you can intentionally soften your chest and take some relaxed, deep breaths. This will help you look at his point of view and find a way to agree with him. You may be surprised at the results!

THE LANGUAGE OF LOVE

What does it mean to embody compassion? Dozens of books from every spiritual tradition exhort us to live compassionately. "Love your neighbor as yourself" is easily said, but what does that mean? Just type the word *self-esteem* into Google and you will find hundreds of pages defining self-esteem as anything from material wealth to Buddhahood. By learning to observe your body language you can begin to identify the postures of not loving yourself. I believe this is the first step toward developing a compassionate stance that can improve our connection to others. Paul Ekman does not qualify compassion or love as emotions. He called compassion a reaction to an emotion. And because in loving someone we experience many different emotions, including anger and even disgust, while still loving the person, Ekman differentiates love from emotion. Susana Bloch includes tenderness and lust as basic emotions, and includes other manifestations of love in her lexicon of mixed emotions.

We speak of "the look of love," or "a kind demeanor," or "a face you can trust." I mentioned earlier that our brains are able to differentiate between a kind face and cruel one. Whether you can measure and label it or not, we can recognize when someone is acting out of love, selfishness, pity, or fear. Therefore there has to be a posture, an attitude that communicates it. When all else fails, you can simply tilt your head slightly to the side (tenderness), allow your spine to soften (remember the saints), and breathe evenly.

Throughout this book we have looked at different aspects of body language and how they reflect aspects of our self-image. The relationships among the parts of the self give excellent clues to the state of our self-esteem. Studying tension, self-deception, and emotional reactions can begin to paint an accurate picture of your life.

The Bible's exhortation to love your neighbor as yourself is more challenging than it at first appears because it requires you to love yourself first. Before you can love yourself you must know who you are, otherwise you are trying to love a stranger. The more you see about yourself, the more you can begin to understand other people and the more compassion you can have for yourself. This process of listening to your own body language will begin to open you to where others live. For example, how many times a day do you judge yourself? Put yourself down? Or descend from what might have been compassion into self-pity? Each time a self-deprecating thought enters your head, there is an accompanying physical posture. Can you begin to notice that posture and intentionally introduce the language of compassion to your own system? Then, when someone is acting like a jerk or a bore, you can learn how to shift from irritation to compassion. You see the jerk and the bore in yourself, and you blend, mirror, or just sit and breathe. This person then may be able to reveal his true beauty. And even if he can't, if his defenses and conditioning are so deeply etched that he cannot give up these habits, you still will be better off than you would have been if you had reacted in the same old way.

This is not to say that what we tend to call negative emotions are all wrong. Anger, fear, and sadness are important aspects of the human condition, even essential for survival at times. Anger can propel you to accomplish great tasks or protect a loved one.

Sadness invites help when you are bereft. And fear keeps us from jumping off of buildings or entering lions' cages. It is when these emotions interfere with our ability to love ourselves and others that they suck us of vitality.

TOWARD A NEW YOU

When one is pierced by love—whether it be romantic, compassionate empathy, maternal, or sacred, the emotion, as discussed earlier, seems to originate in the torso, Delsarte's emotional zone. But how is it expressed? Can I have a compassionate torso, loving arms, and understanding eyes? How does a compassionate person breathe? What is the rhythm of their gestures? No one would argue that Martin Luther King Jr. was not full of compassion for humanity. Yet he spoke with fire and passion, his words ringing like a clarion call. Was it just his words that touched people? The following exercise may be the most challenging in the book. I never stop learning from it.

There are two ways to experiment with this exercise.

1. Create an intention. If you know you are going to be in a challenging situation— you have to fire someone, deny someone what they have asked of you, or even have a conversation with someone you find irritating—make a decision in advance to try to adjust your body language.
2. If you find yourself in an interaction that is triggering anger, irritation, disgust, or some other emotion that separates you from the person you are engaged with, you can try in the moment to experiment.

You can use any of the tools that have already been listed in this book. Or you can zero in on the emotional parts of the self—the torso, breath, forearms, calves, cheeks, and so on, and notice how you are using them. If you are holding your breath, release it. If you are gripping your calves, allow them to stretch out. If you are thrusting out your chest, soften it. Afterward you can record your observations about the interaction and what took place. You may discover that your anger always begins in the same part of your body. Or that your brusque dismissal of people actually covers a kind of fear inside yourself. Or your impatience with stupidity may become a genuine wish to help someone.

Exploration Checklist

☐ Practice mirroring someone during an interaction.

☐ Explore how you can blend with another person by posturally agreeing with their point of view.

☐ Study your lack of compassion toward yourself. How does it affect your posture, and can you use the language of compassion to alter your own state?

☐ As you work with "Toward a New You," try to observe yourself during a negative interaction and introduce a change in one of your emotional zones in order to invite a compassionate attention.

CONCLUSION

We have spent too many hundreds of years blind to what is right under our noses, and above our noses for that matter. Thanks to a combination of puritanical thought and the mechanistic notion of "I think, therefore I am," we have forgotten this most profound biofeedback system. In fact, biofeedback is a system in which you are hooked up to a machine in order to understand how you are feeling! Why not bypass the middleman (or middle machine) and return to the direct knowledge that has been available for all time? You contain all the secrets of the universe within you—as the Sufis say, it's as close as your jugular vein. As the prevailing mechanistic paradigm shifts to a more holistic view of the organism, we can begin to see the patterns of our postural choices reflected in our relationships, emotional states, and physiological health. As science digs deeper into the subatomic structure of the human organism, we may discover that even our atoms dance in an intentional manner that is reflected in our body language. Certainly we are just at the beginning of this exciting journey that can only lead to a greater understanding of our place in the universe.

APPENDIX:
WORKSHEET FOR
GOAL SETTING

DATE:

GOAL:

EFFORT

    PHYSICAL:

    MENTAL:

    EMOTIONAL:

MOTIVE

    PHYSICAL:

    MENTAL:

    EMOTIONAL:

Comments:

Noticings:

Your goals can be clear plans that you are actively working on (such as finish graduate school, renovate the kitchen) or ongoing wishes that have been with you for years (such as lose forty-five pounds, find a meaningful relationship) or impossible dreams (such as sell my screenplay, get out of debt). You may find that there are several different efforts and motivations at work, so feel free to list them all. The comments can be about anything—a free association. The noticings are an opportunity for you to look at what you've written and reflect on how your words connect with your behavior as well as your body language. Here is an example for two weeks of one goal.

DATE: 4/12

GOAL: Lose 45 pounds

EFFORT

PHYSICAL: Cut calories

MENTAL: Tell myself I don't need all this food

EMOTIONAL: Don't know

MOTIVE

PHYSICAL: Get my blood pressure down; fit into a size 12

MENTAL: I don't know what my thoughts are; I should pay attention

EMOTIONAL: Would like a date once in a while

Comments: I love food, I hate the way I look—hey, wait, isn't that an emotion?

Noticings: I get hungry every day at 3 P.M. It's around the time when things get boring at work . . . and I get hungry about an hour before bed, even after dinner, just sitting there . . . actually, I'm always hungry. The minute I finish a meal I'm thinking about the next one.

DATE: 4/19

GOAL: Lose 45 pounds (ARGH!)

EFFORT

PHYSICAL: It's not so easy to cut calories; I thought it would be easy. Maybe I should work out.

MENTAL: Okay, maybe I should come up with some kind of sentence—you know like, if you didn't eat this cake, you could be gorgeous. Ugh!

EMOTIONAL: This sucks. Just the thought of doing this makes me depressed.

MOTIVE

PHYSICAL: I will be healthier. Well, why don't I want that?

MENTAL: My thoughts are a jumble around this.

EMOTIONAL: I'm scared. What if I try and fail? What if I still don't get any love? What if I'm still ugly?

Comments: Why? Why am I always hungry? Why do I think I'm ugly? Is that a thought or an emotion?

Noticings: Everything I write is negative—hating the way I look, being depressed. My chest is all caved in and three times today I noticed that my fists were clenched. Am I angry at something? And what is that feeling in the pit of my stomach—is it really hunger?

RESOURCES

BOOKS

Gregory S. Aldrete, *Gestures and Acclamations in Ancient Rome* (Baltimore: Johns Hopkins University Press, 1999).

David F. Armstrong, William C. Stokoe, and Sherman E. Wilcox, *Gesture and the Nature of Language* (Cambridge, Massachusetts: Cambridge University Press, 1995).

Alain Berthoz, *The Brain's Sense of Movement* (Cambridge, Massachusetts: Harvard University Press, 2000).

Hyrum Conrad, editor, *The Development of Alba Emoting* (Rexburg, Idaho: Brigham Young University, 2003).

Antonio Damasio, *Descartes' Error* (New York: Avon Books, 1995).

_____. *The Feeling of What Happens* (San Diego: Harcourt, 2000).

Charles Darwin, *The Expression of the Emotions in Man and Animals* (Chicago: University of Chicago Press, 1965).

Isha Schwaller de Lubicz, *The Opening of the Way* (Rochester, Vermont: Inner Traditions, 1981).

Karlfried Graf Durckheim, *Hara: The Vital Center of Man* (Rochester, Vermont: Inner Traditions, 2004).

Ken Dychtwald, *BodyMind* (New York: Tarcher/Putnam, 1986).

Paul Ekman, *Emotions Revealed* (New York: Henry Holt, 2003).

_____. *What the Face Reveals* (New York: Oxford University Press, 1997).

Moshe Feldenkrais, *Awareness Through Movement* (San Francisco: Harper, 1991).

_____. *The Elusive Obvious* (Cupertino, California: Meta Publications, 1981).

_____. *The Potent Self* (Berkeley, California: Frog Ltd., 2002).

Belinda Gore, *Ecstatic Body Postures* (Santa Fe, New Mexico: Bear and Company, 1995).

Henry Gray, *Gray's Anatomy of the Human Body* (Philadelphia: Running Press Books, 1974).

Claude Kipnis, *The Mime Book* (New York: Harper Colophon Books, 1976).

Marc McCutcheon, *The Compass in Your Nose and Other Astonishing Facts About Humans* (Los Angeles: Jeremy P. Tarcher, 1989).

David McNeill, *The Face, A Natural History* (Boston: Little, Brown, 1998).

Candace Pert, *The Molecules of Emotion* (New York: Touchstone, 1997).

Lavinia Plonka, *What Are You Afraid Of? A Body/Mind Guide to Courageous Living* (New York: Tarcher/Penguin, 2005).

Peter Ralston, *Cheng Hsin: The Principles of Effortless Power* (Berkeley, California: North Atlantic Books, 1999).

Agya Rangacharya, *The Natyasastra—English Translation with Critical Notes* (New Delhi, India: Munshiram Manoharial, 2003).

Marshall Rosenberg, *Non-Violent Communication, A Language of Life* (Encinitas, California: Puddle Dancer Press, 2003).

Lisa Sarasohn, *The Woman's Belly Book* (Novato, California: New World Library, 2006).

Genevieve Stebbins, *Delsarte System of Expression* (New York: Werner, 1902, out of print).

Richard Strozzi Heckler, editor, *Aikido and the New Warrior* (Berkeley, California: North Atlantic Books, 1985).

Mabel Todd, *The Thinking Body* (Princeton, New Jersey: Princeton Book Company, 1959).

Thomas Leabhart, ed., *Essays on François Delsarte* (Claremont, California: Mime Journal, 2004).

Frank R. Wilson, *The Hand* (New York: Vintage Press, 1999).

MAGAZINE ARTICLES

Michael Abrams, "Can You See with Your Tongue?" *Discover* magazine, June 2003.

Deborah Blum, "Face It!" *Psychology Today,* September/October 1998.

Richard Conniff, "Reading Faces." *Smithsonian,* January 2004.

Malcom Gladwell, "The Naked Face." *The New Yorker,* December 2002.

Steven Johnson, "Emotions and the Brain: Fear." *Discover*, March 2003.

Fernando Pagés Ruiz, "Symbolic Gestures." *Yoga Journal,* December 2002.

Heather Wax, "See Me, Feel Me: The Twists of Empathy." *Science and Theology News,* February 2004.

ONLINE RESOURCES

Articles

www.accessexcellence.org/WN/SU/lying599.html: Sean Henahan, "The Science of Lying."

www.context.org/ICLIB/IC04/Dobson.htm: Terry Dobson, "Aikido in Action."

www.gutenberg.org/etext/12200: "The Delsarte System of Oratory"—a compilation of various writers, along with some of Delsarte's notes.

www.hearthmath.com: Information on Heart/Head Entrainment—Institute of HeartMath.

www.members.aol.com/nonverbal2/diction1.htm: David Givens, "The Nonverbal Dictionary of Gestures, Signs and Body Language Cues."

WORKSHOPS, RESEARCH, AND PRACTITIONERS

www.albaemotingna.org: Provides basic information on the Alba Emoting Method, workshops, and a list of U.S. certified teachers.

www.DelsarteProject.com: Delsartean philosophy and movement taught by Joe Williams.

www.Feldenkrais.com: Offers information about the Feldenkrais Method and a directory of practitioners and classes in North America.

www.laviniaplonka.com: Workshops in body language and personal development.

www.paulekman.com: Information and workshops related to Paul Ekman's research.

INDEX

ABOUT THE AUTHOR

A former artist in residence for the Guggenheim Museum, Lavinia Plonka has taught workshops and consulted around the globe—from the Irish National Folk Theater to Esalen, and inner-city schools to rehabilitation centers. Her first book, *What Are You Afraid Of? A Body/Mind Guide to Courageous Living,* has been translated into five languages. She is director of the Asheville Movement Center in North Carolina, where she maintains a busy practice.